Talk to your healthcare provider about
your specific dietary restrictions.

THE LOW-FAT SUPERMARKET SHOPPER'S GUIDE

MAKING HEALTHY CHOICES FROM THOUSANDS OF BRAND-NAME FOODS

COMPLETELY REVISED AND UPDATED

JAMIE POPE, M.S., R.D.
MARTIN KATAHN, PH.D.

W. W. NORTON & COMPANY
NEW YORK   LONDON

For information about permission to reproduce selections from this title,
write to Permissions, W. W. Norton & Company, Inc., 500 Fifth Avenue,
New York, NY 10110

Manufacturing by Victor Graphics, Inc.
Book design by Margaret M. Wagner
Production manager: Amanda Morrison

ISBN 0-393-32585-7 pbk.

W. W. Norton & Company, Inc.
500 Fifth Avenue, New York, N.Y. 10110
www.wwnorton.com

W. W. Norton & Company Ltd.
Castle House, 75/76 Wells Street, London W1T 3QT

3 4 5 6 7 8 9 0

INTRODUCTION

Whether your goal is weight loss, weight maintenance, or a wish to reduce your risk of heart disease, certain cancers, and diabetes, this little guide can cut your shopping time for a lower-fat and more nutritious diet in half.

We have examined thousands of brand name foods and, in this *Supermarket Shopper's Guide*, we bring you the most recently available data on their total fat, saturated fat, carbohydrate, total calories, dietary fiber, and sodium content. In addition, we present guidelines for how to make healthful choices in each section of the grocery store—e.g., bread, meat, frozen dishes, etc.—which apply to both weight management and disease prevention. Take some time to study this guide, make up a shopping list, and you will save hours standing in the aisles of your grocery store. (Cholesterol content for commonly consumed foods will be found in Appendix A, pages 117–18.)

DISEASE PREVENTION

All major organizations agree that too much fat is the greatest health hazard in the average American's diet. The single most positive step you can take, from a nutritional standpoint, to reduce your risk of heart disease, certain forms of cancer, obesity, and obesity-related degenerative diseases is to reduce the fat in your diet. Indeed, overconsumption of saturated fat is the dietary factor most associated with high blood cholesterol, which is a major risk factor for heart disease.

Studies have shown that people underestimate their fat consumption from between 20 percent to almost as much as 50 percent! On average, Americans consume almost 40 percent of their calories from fat. The American Heart Association recommends that this be reduced to between 20 percent and 30 percent, while many health experts suggest that the lower end of the range is most desirable. Thus, this recommendation turns out to match that for weight loss and maintenance.

WEIGHT LOSS AND MAINTENANCE

Any "diet" that will temporarily help you reduce calorie intake below energy expenditure will lead to weight loss. The real problem occurs after weight loss. That's because the vast majority of weight losers find that maintaining a weight loss is much more difficult than losing weight in the first place.

Persons who have lost significant amounts of weight on various diets **and, in addition, are able to claim permanent success in the years that follow** have something in common. On average, they report that in maintaining their weight loss, they have cut their fat consumption to around 25 percent of total calories. For most women, this means about 50 grams of fat a day for an 1,800-calorie diet and, for men, about 60 grams of fat a day for approximately 2,200 calories.

Successful people report that the two most effective ways to make sure they remain successful are monitoring their calorie intake, or their fat intake, or both.

Health experts agree that **the healthiest way to lose weight** is with a well-balanced diet that includes foods from all the food groups. If you eliminate healthful plant foods from your diet for long periods of time (grains, fruits, and vegetables) you may actually be depriving your body of vitamins, minerals, fiber, and thousands of other phytochemicals that help prevent heart disease and certain forms of cancer. For weight loss, we recommend a moderately low-fat diet of between 20 to 50 grams of fat per day for a woman on a diet of 1,200 calories, and for men, between 30 and 60 grams of fat on a diet of around 1,800 calories. In addition, to facilitate weight and appetite control, the majority of your daily carbohydrate choices should include vegetables, fruits, beans, and grain-based foods that are minimally processed, rich in fiber, and low in refined flour and sugar.

HOW TO USE THIS GUIDE

Keep track of the items you choose from this food guide, along with any others that you may have chosen at the supermarket **that meet the guidelines** we have suggested for each category of food. The guidelines are summarized on pages 9–15. They also appear at the beginning of the list of each category of food throughout the guide. The guidelines are especially important when you choose regional or store brands, rather than the national brands included in the guide. However, since regional and store brands are often actually produced by the major national processors under different labels, the nutritional values of these foods will generally be similar to those we list for the national brands. You can also refer to the listing in Appendix B on pages 119–28 of Web sites for over

100 food companies to find nutrition information for new food products or products not included in this guide.

DESIGNING A HEALTHFUL DIET: USING FOOD LABELS

The food label reproduced on the following page is required on all processed foods. Do not be misled by the "% Daily Value," which is based on a daily diet of 2,000 calories. It suggests 65 grams of fat, which, with 2,000 calories, may be too high for the average woman and may lead to weight gain.

HOW TO FIND THE INFORMATION YOU WANT IN THE DIFFERENT FOOD CATEGORIES

A list of the product categories in this guide begins on page 19. The specific food products are listed alphabetically within each category, or, when there are subcategories, within each subcategory.

For example, the list of BREADS begins on page 36. There are many subcategories, such as loaf breads, variety breads, sandwich buns, etc., within the bread group. Thus the various bread products are listed in alphabetical order within each subcategory in these groups.

ABBREVIATIONS USED IN THIS BOOK

<	less than
≤	less than or equal to
cal.	calories
fiber g.	dietary fiber grams
~	about, or roughly
w/	with
w/o	without
avg.	average values
prep	prepared
f/	from
fzn	frozen

Nutrition Facts

Serving Size ½ cup (114g)
Servings Per Container 4

Amount Per Serving

Calories 90   Calories from Fat 30

	% Daily Value*
Total Fat 3g	**5%**
Saturated Fat 0g	**0%**
Cholesterol 0mg	**0%**
Sodium 300mg	**13%**
Total Carbohydrate 13g	**4%**
Dietary Fiber 3g	**12%**
Sugars 3g	
Protein 3g	

Vitamin A 80%	•	Vitamin C 60%
Calcium 4%	•	Iron 4%

* Percent Daily Values are based on a 2,000 calorie diet. Your daily values may be higher or lower depending on your calorie needs:

	Calories:	2,000	2,500
Total Fat	Less than	65g	80g
Sat Fat	Less than	20g	25g
Cholesterol	Less than	300mg	300mg
Sodium	Less than	2,400mg	2,400mg
Total Carbohydrate		300g	375g
Dietary Fiber		25g	30g

Calories per gram:
Fat 9 • Carbohydrate 4 • Protein 4

6

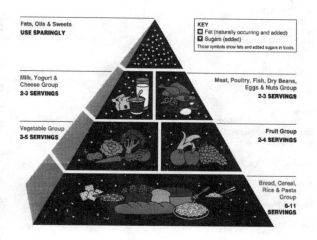

Use the U.S.D.A. FOOD GUIDE PYRAMID to form the basis for your overall diet. Since a plant-based diet affords the greatest nutritional protection against heart disease and certain cancers, we recommend that you chose a majority of foods (55 to 60 percent of calories) from the two lowest levels of the pyramid, i.e., whole-grain foods, vegetables, and fruits. A total of 9 servings from the combined fruit and vegetable groups is better than just 5! Choose low-fat dairy products and lean cuts of meat. Replace some of the animal protein from meat with beans, soy products, and nuts. Proposed changes to the pyramid include greater emphasis on whole grains and "healthy" fats as found in fish, nuts, and olive oil.

SELECTION GUIDELINES AND TIPS

The tips provide suggestions to aid in weight management, as well as how to increase the nutritional and disease-prevention value of selections within each food group.

Produce
FRUITS
1 gram fat or less per serving (½ cup or 140 grams)
Tips: Fruit is an excellent low-fat choice **anytime**. Generally choose fresh fruit, or if not available or suitable for a recipe, use canned or frozen packed in juice or "lite" syrup.

VEGETABLES
1 gram fat or less per serving (½ cup or 85 grams)
Tips: Vegetables (along with fruits) are rich sources of vitamins, minerals, fiber, and

thousands of recently discovered phytochemicals that may help protect against cancers and heart disease. These chemicals are often represented by different colors, so eat a wide variety of different-colored vegetables and fruits each day, being sure to frequently include cruciferous vegetables, e.g., broccoli, cauliflower, cabbage, Brussels sprouts.

SALAD BAR
Prepackaged salad makings with one or two servings (4 to approximately 6 ounces in weight) are now available to make it easier to prepare a healthful meal for just one or two persons. Use full-fat salad dressings with care—they may contain 11–13 grams of fat per tablespoon.

Meats
BEEF
3 grams fat or less per 1 ounce cooked (less than 9 grams per 3-ounce serving cooked)
These criteria apply to beef, pork, luncheon meats, cold cuts, meat spreads, frankfurters, sausage, and bacon.
Tips: Choose "lean" (~ 7% fat in raw meat or 10% in cooked weight) or "extra lean" (5% fat in cooked meat). If meats are not labeled as to fat content, choose minimally marbled cuts, trimmed to less than ¼ inch fat.

A 3–4 ounce serving of meat is approximately the size of a deck of cards. Restaurant portions for entrees are generally double this size.

There are many new varieties of low-fat and fat-free luncheon meats and cold cuts. In general, portion sizes will be around 2 ounces. However, the number of slices totaling a serving will vary between brands. Be sure to calculate the amount of fat according to the weight of the number of slices you actually consume.

POULTRY
2 grams fat or less per ounce cooked
Tip: Most of the fat in poultry is around the skin, so it's best to remove it before cooking. Remove it before eating if cooked with skin on.

FISH
2 grams fat or less per ounce cooked
Tips: Include fish several times per week as a replacement for higher-fat meats. Make tuna salad with either low-fat or fat-free mayonnaise, or blend equal parts mayonnaise and yogurt for a dressing.

Breads
Tips: Choose whole-grain breads, rolls, and bagels most of the time. In case there is a preference for white breads in your family, substitute the new fiber-enriched

white breads for regular white bread. Croissants, butter rolls, pastries, doughnuts, biscuits, and yeast rolls are often very high in fat. Commercial muffins have generally been "supersized," so look for the brands listed on pages 39–40.

LOAF BREADS, VARIETY BREADS, SANDWICH BUNS, ROLLS, ENGLISH MUFFINS
1 gram fat or less per ounce (2 grams fat or less—and 2 or more grams fiber for loaf breads—per standard 2-ounce serving)

REFRIGERATED AND FROZEN BREADS, BISCUITS, ROLLS
3 grams fat or less per 2-ounce serving

MUFFINS, PASTRIES, SWEET BREAKFAST BREADS, BREAD MIXES
4 grams fat or less per 2-ounce serving

Pasta/Noodles/Macaroni (including noodle mixes)
4 grams fat or less per serving (2 ounces dry or 1 cup cooked)
Tips: Build meals around pasta with lower-fat tomato-based sauces, vegetables, and smaller portions of meat, poultry, or fish.

Rice/Rice Mixes
2 grams fat or less and more than 2 grams fiber per serving (2 ounces dry or 1 cup cooked)
Tips: Brown rice contains as much as 3 times the fiber of white rice (as much as 4 grams per cup). Packaged rice can be cooked without added fat with little reduction in flavor.

Beans and Peas, Canned
2 grams fat or less per ½-cup serving
Tips: As excellent low-fat sources of protein, fiber, iron, folic acid, and minerals, beans are a good way to reduce animal products in your diet. Serve beans with rice, pasta, or whole-grain bread. For convenience, try canned beans that do not contain pork or other meat (see pages 46–49).

Canned Entrees/Main Dishes
8 grams fat or less per 1-cup serving

Soups, Canned and Mixes
3 grams fat or less and less than 1,000 milligrams sodium per 1-cup serving
Tips: When soup is included at the start of a meal, people tend to take in fewer total calories. So, soup in the diet is an aid to weight management. Most broth-based soups will meet our criterion, as will some "cream of " soups when reconstituted with water or low-fat milk.

Sauces and Gravies, Canned, Jarred, Mixes
4 grams fat or less per serving as sauce for main dish (½ cup)
2 grams fat or less per serving as sauce for side dish (¼ cup)

Baking Mixes
4 grams fat or les per serving
Tips: Many baking mixes can be made satisfactorily with less fat or with a combination of less fat and yogurt, and with egg whites or egg substitute for whole eggs. "Lite" dessert and dessert mixes, while lower in fat, are by no means calorie free!

Frostings
2 grams fat per serving (about 2 tablespoons)

Puddings, Pie Fillings, and Gelatins
3 grams fat or less per ½-cup serving
Tip: Use skim or 1% milk for pudding mixes. This trims 15 to 30 calories and 2 to 4 grams of fat off the product's whole-milk nutrition labeling content for each ½-cup serving of the final product.

Cereals (with added fiber criterion)
READY TO EAT
2 grams fat or less, and more than 2 grams fiber, per serving
Tips: Cereals are naturally very low in fat (with the exception of most granolas) and are a great way to add fiber, vitamins, and minerals to your diet. People who have ready-to-eat cereals for breakfast tend to have a more nutritious diet that is lower in fat and cholesterol. Mix high-fiber cereals with those lower in fiber to keep taste and texture interesting. Pay attention to the portion size listed on the nutrition label—many people find that they are accustomed to eating portions two or three times the size on the label.

HOT CEREALS, COOKED WITH WATER
2 grams fat or less, and more than 1 gram fiber, per serving (about 1 cup prepared)
Tip: Remember that adding butter or margarine adds additional fat and calories.

Crackers, Croutons, Bread Sticks
2 grams fat or less per ounce (1 gram fat or less per ½-ounce serving)

Cookies
2 grams fat or less per ounce
Tips: The low-fat cookies listed on pages 76–79 are good choices; just don't

overdo. If overeating cookies is a problem, don't keep them around the house to tempt you.

Packaged Snacks
CHIPS, FRUIT SNACKS, PRETZELS, POPCORN, RICE CAKES
3 grams fat or less per 1-ounce serving
Tips: Choose baked packaged snacks, not fried. Since some baked products are tossed or coated with oil (like bagel chips), check the nutrition label.

CAKES AND PASTRIES
4 grams fat or less per 2-ounce serving

Nutrition/Sports Bars and Shakes
6 grams of fat or less per serving (2-ounce bar or 8-ounce shake)

Candy
1 gram fat or less per 1-ounce serving
Tip: Choosing small, individual packages may help prevent you from overeating, provided you don't take a fistful!

Dairy Foods
Tip: Milk and milk products are an important source of calcium. Women, in particular, should have at least 2 to 3 servings each day, or include other high-calcium or calcium-fortified foods.

MILK
2 grams fat or less per 1 cup (8 ounces)

SOUR CREAM AND CREAM
1 gram fat or less per tablespoon

CHEESES
4 grams fat or less per ounce

YOGURT
2 grams fat or less per cup (8 ounces)

Egg Substitutes
2 grams fat or less per egg equivalent (¼ cup)
Tip: 2 egg whites or ¼ cup egg substitute for 1 whole egg can replace 1 whole egg in most recipes.

Fats

Tips: Many reduced-fat margarines and spreads are now available and can often be acceptable alternatives to full-fat versions. Because these products are generally water based, they are not always useful or comparable to the full-fat versions for cooking and baking. To reduce saturated fat and trans-fat intake, we have found that light olive oil, which contains primarily monounsaturated fat, is a good substitute for butter in many cooking and baking recipes. But remember that all undiluted oils contain approximately 14 grams of fat per tablespoon, and should be used with discretion.

REDUCED-FAT MARGARINES, BUTTER SUBSTITUTES, AND COOKING SPRAYS
6 grams fat or less per tablespoon

REDUCED-FAT MAYONNAISE AND SALAD DRESSINGS
3 grams fat or less per 2-tablespoon serving

Condiments
1 gram fat or less per tablespoon

Frozen Foods

Tip: Portion size and nutrition content vary widely among frozen-food entrees and meals. Keep this in mind when you compare labels and think in terms of the portions you normally eat.

ENTREES
8 grams fat or less and less than 1,000 milligrams sodium per 1-cup serving (minimum 5 ounces)

DINNERS
12 grams fat or less and less than 1,000 milligrams sodium per meal (minimum 10 ounces)

SIDE DISHES/POTATOES
3 grams fat or less per serving (½ cup)

DESSERTS
4 grams fat or less per serving (½ cup or 2-ounce slice)

Miscellaneous (Jellies, Jams, Syrups, Pickles; Hot-Cocoa Mixes)
0 gram fat per serving for jellies, jams, syrups, and pickles
≤ 1 gram fat per cup serving (8 ounces) for hot-cocoa mixes

TO NATIONAL FOOD COMPANIES AND READERS: If you have a product that you feel would be appropriate for inclusion in the next edition of this guide, please send either the label of the product or, if available, complete nutritional information to:

Jamie Pope, M.S., R.D.
Low-Fat Supermarket Shopper's Guide
c/o W. W. Norton & Company
500 Fifth Avenue
New York, NY 10110

ADDENDUM

Sources of Information

The information contained in this guide was obtained from the USDA database, food suppliers and producers directly, company Web sites (see list on pages 119–28), and from standing hours on end in supermarket aisles, reading labels (just as you may be doing now).

Sometimes the values for total fat and saturated fat are available, and listed in the guide, to the nearest tenth of a gram. Sometimes the only information available comes directly from the package label, where it is usually rounded up or down to the nearest .5 gram.

The consumer should be aware that nutritional values obtained from scientific analyses are averages of several food samples, and that individual samples can vary 20 or even 30 percent from each other. Thus an actual serving of a food may actually vary that much from the listing in this guide. So, in truth, it is virtually impossible to keep an absolutely perfect record of your intake. Over time, repeated consumption of the same food will in all probability have equaled the listed value across servings. For weight loss, women should just keep their fat total between 20 and 40 grams of fat per day (say, 30 on average), men 30 to 50 per day (or about 45 on average).

While Food and Drug Administration (FDA) regulations require that food labels reflect the amount a person might customarily consume per eating occasion, food processors have considerable latitude in what can be considered a standardized portion. This means that the serving size on labels for similar foods may often look different in terms of total weight, quantity, calories, fat, and other nutritional content. You must keep in mind the portion you actually eat in keeping a record!

The FDA regulations require that commonly used terms describing calories, sodium, sugar, fiber, fat, and cholesterol in food must meet the following criteria when used in conjunction with a specific claim for that nutrient:

- *Free:* less than 5 calories; less than 0.5 gram of sugar; less than 5 milligrams of sodium; less than 0.5 gram of fat; less than 5 milligrams of cholesterol and 0.5 gram of saturated fat per serving.

- *Low:* less than 140 milligrams of sodium; less than 40 calories; 3 grams of fat or less per serving size. [1]

- *High:* Benefits the consumer by providing more than 20 percent of the amount recommended for daily eating, as in high fiber.

- *Source of:* Beneficial because it provides 10 to 19 percent of the nutrient recommended to be eaten each day.

- *Reduced or Less:* Both mean at least 25 percent less than the original product in sodium, calories, fat, saturated fat, or cholesterol.

- *Light:* If a product has more than 50 percent calories from fat, light means at least 50 percent reduction in fat. If it has less than 50 percent calories from fat, product can be either 50 percent reduced in fat or have one-third fewer calories.

- *Light in sodium:* Reduces sodium of original product by 50 percent.

We have included information for the twenty most frequently consumed fruits, vegetables, and varieties of fish, as recommended by the FDA, in an effort to make this counter as complete and convenient as possible. (We do not include avocados because they contain about 20 grams of fat per half cup, sliced or cubed.)

The recommended amounts of fat in the preceding Selection Guidelines and Tips, which are repeated at the beginning of each section in this guide, are based on our experience in helping people design a healthful low-fat diet averaging

---

[1] The majority of our criteria meet the FDA's "low-fat" criterion. However, within some categories our criteria are slightly more flexible because of the limited options and to make your diet livable.

about 25 percent of calories from fat. However, whatever your fat-gram goal, you will find a selection of breakfast, lunch, and dinner foods, plus snacks, that will help you meet your target.

RECOMMENDED VALUES

Total fat:	Women 20–50 grams per day
	Men 30–60 grams per day
Saturated fat:	Women 7–17 grams per day
	Men 10–20 grams per day
Carbohydrate:	Women 150–250 grams per day
	Men 175–275 grams per day
Fiber:	25–40 grams per day
Sodium:	2,400 milligrams or less per day

If you are under medical care, have your physician or dietitian individualize recommended levels for your medical profile.

Produce/Fruits

Criterion for general selection ≤ 1 gram fat per serving (¹/₂ cup, 140 grams); canned and frozen varieties packed in fruit juice or "extra lite" syrup

Fresh (most frequently consumed)

	Serving	Total Fat (g)	Saturated Fat (g)	Total Carbohydrate (g)	Total Calories	Dietary Fiber (g)	Sodium (mg)
apple, whole w/peel	1 medium	0.5	0.1	21	81	4	0
banana	1 medium	0.5	0.2	28	109	3	1
cantaloupe	¹/₄ melon	0.0	0.0	12	50	1	25
cherries, sweet	¹/₂ cup	0.7	0.2	12	52	2	0
grapefruit	¹/₂ medium	0.0	0.0	16	60	6	0
grapes, Thompson seedless	¹/₂ cup	0.5	0.2	14	57	1	2
honeydew melon	¹/₄ small	0.3	0.1	22	87	2	25
kiwi fruit	1 medium	0.5	0.0	12	50	2	0
lemon	1 medium	0.0	0.0	5	15	1	5
lime	1 medium	0.0	0.0	7	20	2	0
nectarine	1 medium	0.5	0.0	16	70	2	0
orange	1 medium	0.2	0.0	15	62	3	0
peach	1 medium	0.1	0.0	11	42	2	0
pear	1 medium	0.7	0.0	25	98	4	0
pineapple	1 cup	0.7	0.1	19	76	2	2
plum	1 medium	0.4	0.0	9	36	1	0
strawberries	1 cup	0.5	0.0	10	43	3	2
tangerine	1 medium	0.2	0.0	9	37	2	2
watermelon	1 cup	0.7	0.1	11	49	1	3

Canned

	Serving	Total Fat (g)	Saturated Fat (g)	Total Carbohydrate (g)	Total Calories	Dietary Fiber (g)	Sodium (mg)
Del Monte							
applesauce	¹/₂ cup	0.0	0.0	21	90	1	5
applesauce, unsweetened	¹/₂ cup	0.0	0.0	13	50	2	5
fruit cocktail	¹/₂ cup	0.0	0.0	15	60	1	10
peaches, extra-light syrup	¹/₂ cup	0.0	0.0	14	60	1	10
pear halves, extra-light syrup	¹/₂ cup	0.0	0.0	15	60	1	10
pineapple chunks, in juice	¹/₂ cup	0.0	0.0	17	70	1	10
Dole							
mandarin orange segments	¹/₂ cup	0.0	0.0	19	80	1	10
mixed tropical fruit	¹/₂ cup	0.0	0.0	20	80	1	10
pineapple chunks, in juice	¹/₂ cup	0.0	0.0	15	60	1	10
Mott's natural applesauce	¹/₂ cup	0.0	0.0	14	50	1	0
Musselman's natural applesauce	¹/₂ cup	0.0	0.0	13	50	2	10

	Serving	Total Fat (g)	Saturated Fat (g)	Total Carbohydrate (g)	Total Calories	Dietary Fiber	Sodium (mg)
Dried							
Dole							
prunes, pitted	1/3 cup	0.0	0.0	35	147	3	7
raisins, seedless and golden	1/4 cup	0.0	0.0	31	130	2	10
Sun-Maid/Sunsweet							
apple	1/3 cup	0.0	0.0	36	147	4	360
apricots	5 apricots	0.0	0.0	24	100	4	0
apricot, bits	1/4 cup	0.0	0.0	22	83	2	23
dates, chopped	1/4 cup	0.0	0.0	32	120	3	0
dates, pitted	1/2 cup	0.0	0.0	64	240	6	0
fruit bits, various, avg.	1/4 cup	0.0	0.0	24	91	2	0
mixed fruit, morsels	1/4 cup	0.0	0.0	28	120	2	55
peaches	4 pieces	0.0	0.0	33	147	4	0
pineapple	1/3 cup	0.0	0.0	34	131	1	20
plums	1/3 cup	0.0	0.0	24	91	3	5
tropical mix	1/4 cup	0.8	0.8	24	106	2	34
Produce/Vegetables							
Criterion for general selection ≤ 1 gram fat per 1/2 cup serving							
Fresh (most frequently consumed)							
asparagus, cooked	1/2 cup	0.1	0.1	4	22	1	2
bell pepper, chopped, raw	1/2 cup	0.1	0.0	5	20	1	1
broccoli, cooked	1/2 cup	0.1	0.0	5	26	3	22
cabbage, shredded, cooked	1/2 cup	0.3	0.0	3	17	2	6
carrots, cooked	1/2 cup	0.1	0.0	8	35	3	51
cauliflower, cooked	1/2 cup	0.3	0.0	3	14	2	9
celery, cooked	1/2 cup	0.2	0.0	5	21	1	47
corn, whole kernal, cooked	1/2 cup	1.0	0.2	21	89	2	14
cucumber, w/o skin, sliced	1/2 cup	0.1	0.0	1	7	0	1
green (snap) beens, cooked	1/2 cup	0.2	0.0	5	22	2	2
iceberg lettuce, raw	1 cup	0.1	0.0	1	7	1	5
leaf lettuce, raw	1 cup	0.2	0.0	2	10	1	5
mushrooms, raw	1/2 cup	0.2	0.0	2	12	1	2
onion, green/spring, raw, chopped	1/4 cup	0.1	0.0	2	8	1	4
onion, white, raw, chopped	1/2 cup	0.1	0.0	7	30	1	2
potato, baked, w/skin	1 medium	0.2	0.0	36	160	4	17
potato, sweet, baked w/skin	1 medium	0.1	0.0	28	117	3	11
radishes	5 medium	0.1	0.0	1	5	0	5

	Serving	Total Fat (g)	Saturated Fat (g)	Total Carbohydrate (g)	Total Calories	Dietary Fiber	Sodium (mg)
squash, summer, slices, cooked	½ cup	0.3	0.1	4	18	1	1
tomatoes, raw	1 medium	0.5	0.0	7	35	1	5
Canned							
Contadina							
tomatoes, diced	½ cup	0.0	0.0	6	30	1	200
tomatoes, diced, w/Italian herbs	½ cup	0.0	0.0	10	45	1	470
tomatoes, diced, w/roasted garlic	½ cup	0.0	0.0	10	45	1	560
tomatoes, diced, w/sautéed onion	½ cup	0.0	0.0	9	40	1	300
tomatoes, stewed	½ cup	0.0	0.0	9	35	1	220
Del Monte							
asparagus, spears or tips	½ cup	0.0	0.0	3	20	1	420
beans, green, French style	½ cup	0.0	0.0	4	20	2	390
beans, lima	½ cup	0.0	0.0	15	80	4	390
beets, sliced, pickled	½ cup	0.0	0.0	19	80	2	380
beets, sliced/whole	½ cup	0.0	0.0	8	35	2	290
carrots, sliced	½ cup	0.0	0.0	8	35	3	300
corn, fiesta style	½ cup	1.0	0.0	12	50	2	310
corn, golden, cream style	½ cup	1.0	0.0	20	90	2	360
corn, golden, whole kernel, unsalted	½ cup	1.0	0.0	11	60	3	10
corn, white, cream style	½ cup	1.0	0.0	21	100	2	360
corn, white, whole kernel	½ cup	1.0	0.0	11	60	3	360
mixed vegetables	½ cup	0.0	0.0	8	40	2	360
mixed vegetables, unsalted	½ cup	0.0	0.0	8	40	2	25
peas, sweet	½ cup	0.0	0.0	13	60	4	390
peas, sweet, unsalted	½ cup	0.0	0.0	11	60	4	10
peas, w/carrots	½ cup	0.0	0.0	11	60	2	360
potatoes, new, sliced	½ cup	0.0	0.0	10	45	2	273
sauerkraut	½ cup	0.0	0.0	4	16	4	720
spinach, chopped	½ cup	0.0	0.0	4	30	2	360
squash, zucchini, w/Italian tomato sauce	½ cup	0.0	0.0	7	30	1	490
tomatoes, stewed, original	½ cup	0.0	0.0	9	35	2	360
tomatoes, stewed, unsalted	½ cup	0.0	0.0	9	35	2	50

	Serving	Total Fat (g)	Saturated Fat (g)	Total Carbohydrate (g)	Total Calories	Dietary Fiber	Sodium (mg)
Green Giant							
asparagus, cut or whole spears (avg.)	½ cup	0.0	0.0	3	20	1	420
asparagus, cut spears, 50% less salt	½ cup	0.0	0.0	3	20	1	210
beans, black	½ cup	0.0	0.0	18	100	5	400
beans, green, cut or French (avg.)	½ cup	0.0	0.0	4	20	1	390
beans, green, cut, 50% less salt	½ cup	0.0	0.0	4	20	1	200
beans, kidney, red	½ cup	0.0	0.0	20	110	6	340
beans, pinto	½ cup	0.5	0.0	20	110	5	280
beets, sliced	½ cup	0.0	0.0	8	35	2	260
beets, sliced, w/o added salt	½ cup	0.0	0.0	8	35	2	60
carrots, sliced	½ cup	0.0	0.0	6	25	2	380
carrots, whole baby	½ cup	0.0	0.0	8	35	3	410
corn, cream style	½ cup	0.5	0.0	22	100	1	430
corn, Niblets	½ cup	0.0	0.0	15	71	2	232
corn, Niblets, 50% less salt	½ cup	0.0	0.0	21	91	2	174
corn, Niblets, w/o added salt & sugar	½ cup	0.0	0.0	20	91	3	0
corn, white	⅓ cup	0.5	0.0	16	61	1	222
corn, w/peppers, mexicorn	⅓ cup	0.0	0.0	14	61	2	434
mixed vegetables	⅓ cup	0.0	0.0	12	60	2	460
mushrooms, sliced	½ cup	0.0	0.0	4	30	2	440
peas, early or sweet	½ cup	0.0	0.0	12	60	3	380
peas, sweet, w/carrots or w/onions (avg.)	½ cup	0.0	0.0	11	60	4	460
peas, sweet, 50% less sodium	½ cup	0.0	0.0	11	60	3	195
salad, three bean	½ cup	0.0	0.0	20	90	4	490
vegetables, garden medley	½ cup	0.0	0.0	9	40	2	360
Hunt's							
tomatoes, original, diced	½ cup	0.0	0.0	5	20	1	380
tomatoes, diced, w/basil, garlic, oregano	½ cup	0.0	0.0	6	25	1	530
tomatoes, diced, w/mild green chilies	½ cup	0.0	0.0	6	30	2	360

	Serving	Total Fat (g)	Saturated Fat (g)	Total Carbohydrate (g)	Total Calories	Dietary Fiber	Sodium (mg)
tomatoes, diced, w/roasted garlic	½ cup	0.0	0.0	6	30	1	480
tomatoes, diced in sauce	½ cup	0.0	0.0	7	30	1	430
tomatoes, stewed, no salt added	½ cup	0.0	0.0	9	40	1	30
tomatoes, whole	½ cup	0.0	0.0	4	20	1	190
tomatoes, whole, no salt added	½ cup	0.0	0.0	4	20	1	15
Progresso							
artichokes, hearts	3 pieces	0.0	0.0	18	90	3	720
beans, black	½ cup	1.0	0.0	17	110	7	400
beans, chickpea/garbanzo	½ cup	1.5	0.0	18	110	5	380
peppers, cherry, hot	3 pieces	0.0	0.0	6	30	3	450
squash, zucchini, Italian style	½ cup	2.0	0.0	7	50	2	400
tomatoes, crushed	½ cup	0.0	0.0	8	40	2	190
tomatoes, whole, peeled	½ cup	0.0	0.0	5	25	1	220
Westbrae Natural/Hain-Celestial							
beans, black, organic	½ cup	0.0	0.0	19	100	5	140
beans, chickpea/garbanzo, organic	½ cup	2.0	0.0	18	110	5	140
beans, chili, kidney pinto & black, organic	½ cup	0.0	0.0	19	100	5	150
beans, Great Northern, organic	½ cup	0.0	0.0	19	100	6	140
beans, green, French cut, organic	½ cup	0.0	0.0	4	20	1	370
beans, Jackson Wonder, organic (Heirloom)	½ cup	0.0	0.0	19	100	5	135
beans, kidney, organic	½ cup	0.0	0.0	18	100	5	140
beans, pinto, organic	½ cup	0.0	0.0	19	100	7	140
beans, red, organic	½ cup	0.0	0.0	19	100	7	140
beans, runner, scarlet, organic (Heirloom)	½ cup	0.0	0.0	20	100	7	140
beans, salad mix, organic	½ cup	0.5	0.0	19	100	5	150
beans, soldier, European, organic (Heirloom)	½ cup	0.0	0.0	16	90	5	140
beans, trout, organic (Heirloom)	½ cup	0.0	0.0	18	100	6	140

	Serving	Total Fat (g)	Saturated Fat (g)	Total Carbohydrate (g)	Total Calories	Dietary Fiber	Sodium (mg)
chili, black beans, spicy, vegetarian, fat-free	1/2 cup	0.0	0.0	15	120	7	160
chili, w/3 beans, mild, vegetarian, fat-free	1/2 cup	0.0	0.0	15	120	7	160
corn, golden, whole kernel, organic	1/2 cup	1.0	0.0	14	90	2	340
corn, white, whole kernel, organic	1/2 cup	1.0	0.0	20	100	1	340
lentils, black beluga, organic	1/2 cup	0.0	0.0	16	100	4	120
peas, sweet, organic	1/2 cup	0.0	0.0	10	60	3	360
soybeans, organic	1/2 cup	7.0	1.0	11	150	3	140
Frozen							
Bird's Eye							
asparagus, spears	8 spears	0.2	0.0	4	21	1	3
beans, green, cut	1/2 cup	0.1	0.0	6	25	2	3
beans, Italian	1/2 cup	0.1	0.0	8	33	3	3
broccoli, chopped	1/2 cup	0.3	0.1	7	36	3	22
broccoli, stir fry	1/2 cup	0.3	0.0	4	26	2	26
broccoli, w/carrots & water chestnuts	1/2 cup	0.2	0.1	7	29	3	32
broccoli, w/corn & red pepper	1/2 cup	0.5	0.1	12	54	3	15
carrots, baby, whole	1/2 cup	0.2	0.0	9	40	2	44
carrots, sliced	1/2 cup	0.2	0.0	9	36	3	44
corn, cob, big ears	2 ears	2.0	0.0	57	238	7	7
corn, sweet	1/2 cup	0.7	0.1	20	83	3	3
dinner, stir fry, Chinese veg.	1/2 cup	0.3	0.1	9	44	3	302
mixed vegetables	1/2 cup	0.5	0.1	17	79	4	56
peas, green	1/2 cup	0.5	0.1	13	71	5	125
peas, green, w/pearl onions	1/2 cup	0.4	0.1	15	77	5	475
spinach, chopped	1/2 cup	0.4	0.1	5	30	2	120
vegetables, Japanese style, stir fry	1/2 cup	0.3	0.1	7	35	2	439
vegetables, pepper style, stir fry	1/2 cup	0.2	0.0	4	15	1	9

	Serving	Total Fat (g)	Saturated Fat (g)	Total Carbohydrate (g)	Total Calories	Dietary Fiber	Sodium (mg)
Green Giant							
carrots, baby, cut, select	½ cup	0.0	0.0	5	20	2	27
corn, cream style	½ cup	1.0	0.0	23	110	2	330
peas, June, early, w/mushrooms (Le Seuer)	½ cup	0.0	0.0	7	40	3	70
peas, sugar snap, select	½ cup	0.0	0.0	5	23	2	0
spinach, leaf, cut	½ cup	0.0	0.0	2	17	2	43
American Mixtures							
broccoli, carrots, cauliflower, skillet	½ cup	0.0	0.0	3	19	2	23
broccoli, carrots, water chestnuts, stir fry	½ cup	0.0	0.0	4	19	2	23
Harvest Fresh							
asparagus, cut	1 cup	0.0	0.0	6	38	2	129
beans, green, w/almonds	½ cup	2.3	0.0	4	45	2	72
beans, lima	½ cup	0.0	0.0	15	80	4	130
broccoli, cauliflower, carrots	½ cup	0.0	0.0	3	15	2	63
broccoli, cut	½ cup	0.0	0.0	3	19	2	114
carrots, baby, cut	½ cup	0.0	0.0	4	15	2	53
corn, Niblets	½ cup	0.4	0.0	13	61	2	45
corn, white	½ cup	0.5	0.0	14	70	2	45
mixed vegetables	½ cup	0.0	0.0	8	38	2	95
peas, sweet	½ cup	0.0	0.0	10	45	3	152
peas, sweet, w/pearl onions	½ cup	0.0	0.0	10	50	3	170
spinach	½ cup	0.0	0.0	3	25	2	240
Ore-Ida							
corn, cob, gold, mini	1 cob	1.0	0.0	16	90	2	0
onion, chopped	½ cup	0.0	0.0	4	19	5	7
vegetables, stew style	½ cup	0.0	0.0	8	38	0	38

Meats/Beef

Criteria for general selection: ≤ 3 grams fat per 1 ounce cooked (≤ 9 grams per 3 ounces cooked); "lean" cuts represent ~ 7% fat in raw meat and 10% in cooked weight, "extra lean" represents 5% fat in cooked meat; select cuts with minimal marbling and fat trimmed to ≤ ¼"

Fresh, Cooked, w/o Added Fat

	Serving	Total Fat (g)	Saturated Fat (g)	Total Carbohydrate (g)	Total Calories	Dietary Fiber	Sodium (mg)
arm/pot roast, lean	3 oz.	7.0	2.6	0	184	0	56
bottom round roast, lean	3 oz.	7.0	2.4	0	178	0	43

	Serving	Total Fat (g)	Saturated Fat (g)	Total Carbohydrate (g)	Total Calories	Dietary Fiber	Sodium (mg)
flank steak, London broil, lean	3 oz.	8.1	3.7	0	176	0	71
ground, extra lean (raw)	3 oz.	4.5	1.5	0	130	0	65
rib steak, lean	3 oz.	9.5	3.8	0	188	0	59
round eye roast, lean	3 oz.	4.2	1.5	0	143	0	53
shank, lean	3 oz.	5.4	2.0	0	171	0	54
sirloin strip steak, lean	3 oz.	8.0	3.1	0	176	0	58
top round steak, lean	3 oz.	4.2	1.4	0	153	0	52
top sirloin steak, lean	3 oz.	6.1	2.4	0	166	0	56
Canned, Cooked							
Libby's roast beef, w/gravy	⅔ cup	3.0	1.5	2	141	0	808

Meats/Pork

Criteria for general selection: ≤ 3 grams fat per 1 ounce cooked (≤ 9 grams per 3 ounces cooked); "lean" cuts represent ~ 7% fat in raw meat and 10% in cooked weight; "extra lean" represents 5% fat in cooked meat; select cuts with minimal marbling and fat trimmed to ≤ ¹/₄"

Fresh, Cooked, w/o Added Fat	Serving	Total Fat (g)	Saturated Fat (g)	Total Carbohydrate (g)	Total Calories	Dietary Fiber	Sodium (mg)
center loin chop, lean	3 oz.	6.9	2.5	0	172	0	51
roast, center loin, lean	3 oz.	7.7	2.8	0	169	0	56
sirloin chop, lean	3 oz.	5.7	1.9	0	164	0	48
tenderloin, lean	3 oz.	4.1	1.4	0	140	0	48
top loin chop, lean	3 oz.	6.6	2.3	0	173	0	55
Hormel/Always Tender							
loin fillets, lemon garlic	3 oz.	3.6	1.2	2	100	0	502
tenderloin, peppercorn	3 oz.	3.2	1.0	2	94	0	505
tenderloin, teriyaki	3 oz.	2.6	0.9	4	101	0	351
Hams							
cured center slice, country style, lean (raw)	3 oz.	7.1	2.4	0	166	0	2292
cured ham, lean, 7% fat, canned	3 oz.	7.2	2.4	0	142	0	908
cured steak, extra lean (before heating)	3 oz.	3.7	1.2	0	104	0	1079
Bryan Foods							
hickory smoked, slice	3 oz.	3.5	1.2	1	92	0	701
smoked, diced	3 oz.	5.0	1.5	0	100	0	930
smoked, 96% fat-free, slice	3 oz.	2.5	1.0	1	90	0	1070
Hormel							
Cure 81	3 oz.	3.1	1.0	0	90	0	883

	Serving	Total Fat (g)	Saturated Fat (g)	Total Carbohydrate (g)	Total Calories	Dietary Fiber	Sodium (mg)
Oscar Mayer							
cured, avg. various styles, slice	3 oz.	3.2	1.1	1	88	0	1146
cured, 96% fat-free, low sodium	3 oz.	3.0	1.1	2	92	0	706

Meats/Miscellaneous

Criteria for general selection: ≤ 3 grams fat per 1 ounce cooked (≤ 9 grams per 3 ounces cooked); "lean" cuts represent ~ 7% fat in raw meat and 10% in cooked weight, "extra lean" represents 5% fat in cooked meat; select cuts with minimal marbling and fat trimmed to ≤ 1/4"

	Serving	Total Fat (g)	Saturated Fat (g)	Total Carbohydrate (g)	Total Calories	Dietary Fiber	Sodium (mg)
Beefalo	3 oz.	5.4	2.3	0	160	0	70
Frog legs	4 legs	0.9	0.2	0	212	0	168
Lamb							
leg, shank, lean	3 oz.	5.7	2.0	0	153	0	56
loin chop, lean	3 oz.	8.3	3.0	0	184	0	71
shoulder, blade chop, lean	3 oz.	9.6	3.4	0	180	0	75
Organ Meats							
brains, beef, raw	3 oz.	7.9	1.8	0	107	0	88
kidney, beef, cooked	3 oz.	2.9	0.9	1	123	0	114
liver, beef, braised	3 oz.	4.2	1.6	3	137	0	60
liver, calf, braised	3 oz.	5.9	2.2	2	140	0	45
Veal							
arm steak, lean	3 oz.	4.5	1.3	0	171	0	77
blade, lean	3 oz.	5.5	1.5	0	168	0	86
loin chop, lean	3 oz.	5.9	2.2	0	149	0	82
rib chop, lean	3 oz.	6.6	2.2	0	185	0	84
sirloin steak, lean	3 oz.	5.3	2.1	0	143	0	72
Venison	3 oz.	2.7	1.1	0	134	0	46

Meats/Luncheon Type, Cold Cuts, Meat Spreads

Criteria for general selection: ≤ 3 grams fat per 1 ounce (≤ 6 grams per 2-ounce reference amount)

	Serving	Total Fat (g)	Saturated Fat (g)	Total Carbohydrate (g)	Total Calories	Dietary Fiber	Sodium (mg)
Alpine Lace							
cooked ham, 97% fat-free	3 oz.	1.5	0.5	2	25	0	600
honey ham, 97% fat-free	3 oz.	1.5	0.5	2	25	0	600
roast beef, extra lean, 97% fat-free	3 oz.	1.5	0.5	1	40	0	300
turkey breast, fat-free	3 oz.	0.0	0.0	1	25	0	500
Bryan Foods							
ham, 96% fat-free	2 oz.	1.5	0.5	1	60	0	660

	Serving	Total Fat (g)	Saturated Fat (g)	Total Carbohydrate (g)	Total Calories	Dietary Fiber	Sodium (mg)
ham, smoked, deli slices, low fat	3 pieces	0.8	0.3	0	30	0	360
turkey breast, smoked, 99% fat-free	3 pieces	0.8	0.3	1	30	0	340
Carl Buddig and Company							
beef	2 oz.	3.7	1.5	0	79	0	811
chicken	2 oz.	5.7	1.5	0	94	0	541
corned beef	2 oz.	3.9	1.6	1	81	0	761
ham	2 oz.	5.3	1.8	1	92	0	783
turkey	2 oz.	5.1	1.8	1	91	0	621
Foster Farms							
honey turkey breast	2 oz.	1.0	0.0	1	60	0	750
oven-roasted chicken breast	2 slices	1.0	0.0	0	50	0	500
oven-roasted natural turkey breast	2 oz.	1.0	0.0	1	60	0	510
oven-roasted turkey breast	2 slices	2.0	1.0	1	60	0	440
oven-roasted white turkey	2 slices	3.0	0.0	2	70	0	460
smoked turkey	2 slices	1.0	0.0	2	60	0	420
smoked turkey breast	2 oz.	0.5	0.0	0	60	0	340
Healthy Choice/deli meats							
browned chicken breast	2 oz.	1.0	0.5	1	60	0	480
chicken breast	2 oz.	1.0	0.5	1	50	0	470
chicken breast, mesquite smoked	2 oz.	1.0	0.5	1	60	0	440
ham	2 oz.	1.5	0.5	1	50	0	480
ham, honey cured	2 oz.	1.5	0.5	2	60	0	480
ham, honey maple flavor	2 oz.	1.5	0.5	2	60	0	480
ham, smoked	2 oz.	1.5	0.5	2	60	0	460
ham, Virginia Brand	2 oz.	1.5	0.5	1	60	0	480
roast beef, medium, or Italian Style	2 oz.	1.5	1.0	1	60	0	480
turkey breast, honey roasted & smoked	2 oz.	1.0	0.5	1	60	0	480
turkey breast, mesquite smoked	2 oz.	1.0	0.5	2	60	0	480
turkey breast, southwest grill	2 oz.	1.0	0.5	1	60	0	480
turkey breast, smoked	2 oz.	1.0	0.5	1	50	0	480

	Serving	Total Fat (g)	Saturated Fat (g)	Total Carbohydrate (g)	Total Calories	Dietary Fiber	Sodium (mg)
Healthy Choice/sliced, packaged meats							
bologna	2 slices	3.0	1.0	7	80	0	480
chicken breast, honey roasted and smoked	4 slices	1.5	0.5	4	70	0	450
chicken breast, oven roasted, or smoked	4 slices	1.5	0.5	3	60	0	450
ham, honey maple	4 slices	1.5	0.5	3	60	0	450
ham, various flavors: baked, Virginia Brand, smoked, mesquite, oven roasted	4 slices	1.5	0.5	2	60	0	450
turkey, honey roasted and smoked	4 slices	1.5	0.5	3	60	0	450
turkey, various flavors: smoked breast and white meat, rotisserie seasoned, oven roasted, mesquite	4 slices	1.5	0.5	2	60	0	450
Libby's Spreadables							
chicken salad	2 oz.	5.3	1.1	6	82	0	265
ham salad	1/3 cup	4.0	1.0	9	100	1	467
Louis Rich (# serving slices = ~ 2 oz.)							
Carving Board meats							
chicken breast classic baked/grill	2 slices	0.2	0.1	2	44	0	514
turkey breast, smoked	2 slices	0.5	0.3	1	42	0	540
cold cuts							
chicken, white, oven roasted	2 slices	3.2	0.8	1	72	0	335
turkey breast w/white turkey, oven roasted	2 slices	1.2	0.3	2	55	0	270
turkey breast, w/white turkey, smoked	2 slices	1.3	0.3	1	56	0	257
turkey ham	2 slices	2.4	0.6	1	63	0	631
turkey, honey roasted, fat-free	2 slices	0.4	0.1	3	57	0	661
turkey, oven roasted, fat-free	2 slices	0.4	0.1	1	50	0	659
turkey salami, or cotto salami	2 slices	5.3	1.6	0	42	0	542

	Serving	Total Fat (g)	Saturated Fat (g)	Total Carbohydrate (g)	Total Calories	Dietary Fiber	Sodium (mg)
Oscar Mayer (# serving slices = ~ 2 oz.)							
bologna, fat-free	2 slices	0.4	0.1	3	44	0	547
chicken breast, honey glazed	4 slices	0.8	0.2	2	57	0	748
chicken breast, oven roasted, fat-free	4 slices	0.3	0.1	1	44	0	646
ham, baked, 96% fat-free	3 slices	2.2	0.5	1	66	0	782
ham, boiled	3 slices	2.3	0.8	1	66	0	849
ham, chopped w/natural juice	2 slices	6.2	2.3	2	101	0	699
ham, honey	3 slices	2.2	0.8	2	70	0	786
ham, smoked	3 slices	2.3	0.8	0	62	0	765
ham, smoked, fat-free	2 slices	0.2	0.1	1	96	0	347
turkey breast, smoked, fat-free	4 slices	0.3	0.1	2	42	0	569
Smart Deli/vegetarian (Lightlife Foods)							
country ham	4 slices	0.0	0.0	5	90	1	400
old-world bologna	4 slices	0.0	0.0	3	70	2	400
roast turkey	4 slices	0.0	0.0	4	80	1	560
three-peppercorn pastrami	4 slices	0.0	0.0	1	60	0	400
Tyson (# serving slices = ~ 2 oz.)							
boxed lunch meats							
cooked ham	5 slices	1.5	0.5	0	60	0	760
honey ham	5 slices	1.5	0.5	1	60	0	760
honey-roasted chicken breast	5 slices	1.0	0.0	3	60	0	590
honey-roasted turkey breast	5 slices	1.0	0.0	4	50	0	590
oven-roasted chicken breast	5 slices	1.0	0.0	2	50	0	590
oven-roasted turkey breast	5 slices	1.0	0.0	0	50	0	590
rotisserie-flavor chicken breast	5 slices	1.0	0.0	2	50	0	590
smoked chicken breast	5 slices	1.0	0.0	1	50	0	590
resealable bag lunch meats (# slices = ~ 1.5 ounces)							
cooked ham	2 slices	1.5	0.5	0	50	0	740
honey ham	2 slices	1.5	0.5	1	50	0	740
honey-roasted chicken breast	2 slices	1.0	0.0	3	45	0	530

	Serving	Total Fat (g)	Saturated Fat (g)	Total Carbohydrate (g)	Total Calories	Dietary Fiber	Sodium (mg)
oven-roasted chicken breast	2 slices	0.5	0.0	1	45	0	530
oven-roasted turkey breast	2 slices	0.5	0.0	1	40	0	560
smoked chicken breast	2 slices	0.5	0.0	1	45	0	530
shaved lunch meats (# slices = ~ 2 oz.)							
cooked ham	3 slices	1.5	0.5	0	60	0	760
honey ham	3 slices	1.5	0.5	1	60	0	760
honey-roasted turkey breast	3 slices	1.0	0.0	4	60	0	640
oven-roasted chicken breast	3 slices	1.0	0.0	2	60	0	640
oven-roasted turkey breast	3 slices	1.0	0.0	2	60	0	640
rotisserie flavor chicken breast	3 slices	1.0	0.0	2	60	0	640
self-serve deli meats (# slices = ~ 2 oz.)							
Black Forest smoked ham	2 slices	2.0	1.0	0	60	0	600
brown sugar ham	2 slices	2.0	1.0	1	70	0	560
corned beef	2 slices	2.0	1.0	0	70	0	530
golden roasted chicken breast	3 slices	1.0	0.0	1	60	0	620
golden roasted turkey breast	2 slices	0.0	0.0	2	70	0	880
hickory smoked turkey breast	2 slices	0.0	0.0	1	70	0	940
honey-cured ham	2 slices	2.0	1.0	2	70	0	500
honey smoked turkey breast	2 slices	0.0	0.0	5	70	0	880
pastrami	2 slices	2.0	1.0	0	70	0	530
roast beef	2 slices	2.0	1.0	1	90	0	710
slow-cured cooked ham	2 slices	2.0	1.0	0	70	0	760
smoked chicken breast	3 slices	1.0	0.0	1	60	0	620
Virginia-brand ham	2 slices	2.0	0.0	0	60	0	600
Worthington Foods/vegetarian (Kellogg's)							
meatless bologna	3 slices	3.0	0.5	3	80	2	660
meatless salami	3 slices	7.0	1.0	3	120	2	800
meatless ham	3 slices	7.0	1.0	3	110	0	400
Yves Veggie Cuisine/vegetarian (Hain-Celestial)							
veggie bologna	4 slices	1.0	0.0	4	0	1	430

	Serving	Total Fat (g)	Saturated Fat (g)	Total Carbohydrate (g)	Total Calories	Dietary Fiber (g)	Sodium (mg)
veggie ham	4 slices	0.0	0.0	6	0	1	480
veggie salami	4 slices	0.0	0.0	5	0	1	390
veggie turkey	4 slices	2.0	0.0	4	0	2	410

Meats/Franks

Criteria for general selection: ≤ 3 grams fat per ounce (≤ 6 grams per 2 ounce serving)

	Serving	Total Fat (g)	Saturated Fat (g)	Total Carbohydrate (g)	Total Calories	Dietary Fiber (g)	Sodium (mg)
Healthy Choice							
low-fat beef franks	1 frank	2.5	1.0	5	70	0	440
low-fat w/turkey, pork, beef	1 frank	2.5	1.0	7	70	0	440
Hebrew National							
beef franks, 97% fat-free	1 frank	1.5	1.0	3	45	0	400
Loma Linda/vegetarian							
corn dog	1 frank	4.0	0.5	22	150	3	500
Louis Rich							
franks, turkey and chicken	1 frank	6.1	1.7	2	85	0	511
Morningstar Farms/vegetarian							
corn dog	1 frank	6.0	1.0	22	170	3	530
Natural Touch/vegetarian							
corn dog	1 frank	6.0	1.0	22	170	3	530
Oscar Mayer							
wieners (beef franks, fat-free)	1 frank	0.3	0.1	3	39	0	464
wieners (fat-free hot dogs)	1 frank	0.3	0.1	2	37	0	487
Yves Veggie Cuisine/vegetarian (Hain-Celestial)							
the good dog	1 frank	1.7	0.1	2	77	1	380
tofu dogs	1 frank	0.5	0.0	2	47	0	241
veggie dogs	1 frank	0.1	0.0	1	56	1	399
veggie dogs, hot 'n' spicy chili	1 frank	1.1	0.1	3	74	2	395
veggie dogs, jumbo	1 frank	1.3	0.3	7	104	2	480

Meats/Sausage and Bacon

Criteria for general selection: ≤ 3 grams fat per ounce

	Serving	Total Fat (g)	Saturated Fat (g)	Total Carbohydrate (g)	Total Calories	Dietary Fiber (g)	Sodium (mg)
Butterball							
turkey sausage, brown and serve, cooked	2 oz.	5.8	1.6	6	112	0	346
Hormel							
Canadian bacon	2 oz.	2.8	1.0	1	68	0	569

	Serving	Total Fat (g)	Saturated Fat (g)	Total Carbohydrate (g)	Total Calories	Dietary Fiber	Sodium (mg)
Louis Rich							
breakfast sausage links	3 links	3.0	1.0	3	70	0	480
breakfast sausage patties	3 patties	3.0	1.0	3	70	0	480
low-fat sausage kielbasa	2 oz.	2.5	1.0	6	80	0	480
smoked sausage	1 pieces	2.5	1.0	6	80	0	480
turkey smoked sausage	2 oz.	5.5	1.5	2	90	0	530
Morningstar Farms/vegetarian							
veggie breakfast sausage links	2 links	3.0	0.5	3	80	0	320
veggie breakfast sausage patties	1 patty	3.0	0.5	3	80	0	270
Natural Touch/vegetarian							
breakfast patty w/organic soy	1 patty	3.0	0.5	4	80	0	250

Poultry

Criterion for general selection: ≤ 2 grams fat per ounce cooked

Fresh, Roasted w/o added fat

	Serving	Total Fat (g)	Saturated Fat (g)	Total Carbohydrate (g)	Total Calories	Dietary Fiber	Sodium (mg)
chicken breast, w/o skin	3 oz.	3.0	0.9	0	140	0	63
chicken drumstick, w/o skin	1 leg	2.5	0.7	0	76	0	42
chicken, light meat, w/o skin	3 oz.	3.5	0.9	0	130	0	43
chicken, thigh, w/o skin	1 thigh	5.7	1.6	0	109	0	46
turkey, dark meat, w/o skin	3 oz.	3.7	1.2	0	138	0	67
turkey, light meat, w/o skin	3 oz.	2.7	0.9	0	134	0	54
Banquet chicken							
nuggets, breast meat, frozen, cooked	1 piece	2.9	0.7	2	40	0	71
patty, breast meat, honey bbq, grilled	1 patty	5.0	2.0	3	110	0	440
Banquet tenders							
breast meat, fat-free, baked	1 piece	0.0	0.0	5	40	1	160
breast meat, w/o skin & bone, frozen, cooked	1 piece	5.0	1.2	5	83	0	160
Butterball chicken breasts							
Italian herb, crispy, baked	1 piece	6.0	2.0	16	190	1	710
lemon pepper, crispy, baked	1 piece	7.0	3.0	16	200	1	420
original, crispy, baked	1 piece	6.0	2.0	16	180	1	500
Butterball chicken tenders							
breast, baked	1 piece	2.3	0.8	6	64	0	154

	Serving	Total Fat (g)	Saturated Fat (g)	Total Carbohydrate (g)	Total Calories	Dietary Fiber	Sodium (mg)
hickory smoked, w/sauce, grilled	1 piece	1.3	0.4	3	40	0	143
Oriental, w/sauce, grilled, cooked	1 piece	1.3	0.5	3	40	0	140
Country Skillet chicken							
chunks, cooked from frozen	1 piece	3.2	0.6	4	54	0	144
tenders, breast, cooked from frozen	1 piece	4.7	1.3	5	80	0	150
Foster Farms chicken tenders							
frozen, raw	1 piece	0.5	0.0	0	40	0	143
99% fat-free, raw	1 piece	0.1	0.0	0	28	0	13
Healthy Choice chicken							
breast, country glaze, frozen	1 piece	5.0	2.0	31	250	3	600
Swanson							
chicken, white meat, premium chunk, canned	2 oz.	1.0	0.5	1	60	0	229
turkey, chunky, premium, white meat, canned	2 oz.	1.8	0.5	4	82	1	201
Tyson chicken							
breast, fillet, marinated	2 oz.	1.2	0.4	0	58	0	136

Fish

Criterion for general selection: ≤ 2 grams fat per ounce cooked

Fresh (USDA's "most frequently consumed varieties")

	Serving	Total Fat (g)	Saturated Fat (g)	Total Carbohydrate (g)	Total Calories	Dietary Fiber	Sodium (mg)
catfish, farmed	3.5 oz.	8.0	1.8	0	151	0	79
catfish, wild	3.5 oz.	2.9	0.7	0	104	0	50
clams, raw, large	5 clams	1.0	0.1	3	74	0	56
cod (Atlantic/Pacific avg.)	3.5 oz.	0.9	0.2	0	104	0	84
crab, blue, canned, drained, cup	½ cup	0.8	0.2	0	67	0	225
flounder/sole	3.5 oz.	1.5	0.4	0	116	0	104
haddock	3.5 oz.	0.9	0.2	0	111	0	86
halibut, Atlantic/Pacific	3.5 oz.	2.9	0.4	0	139	0	68
lobster, northern	3.5 oz.	0.6	0.1	1	97	0	377
lobster, spiny	3.5 oz.	1.9	0.3	3	141	0	226
mackerel, Pacific & jack	3.5 oz.	8.6	2.5	0	171	0	94
ocean perch, Atlantic	3.5 oz.	2.1	0.3	0	120	0	95
orange roughy	3.5 oz.	0.9	0.0	0	88	0	80
oysters, raw, medium size	6 each	2.1	0.7	3	57	0	177
pollock, Atlantic	3.5 oz.	1.3	0.2	0	117	0	109

	Serving	Total Fat (g)	Saturated Fat (g)	Total Carbohydrate (g)	Total Calories	Dietary Fiber	Sodium (mg)
rockfish	3.5 oz.	2.0	0.5	0	120	0	76
scallops (steamed, baked, broiled, avg.)	3.5 oz.	3.5	0.6	3	107	0	208
shrimp, boiled, large	8 pieces	0.5	0.1	0	44	0	99
trout, rainbow, farmed	3.5 oz.	7.1	2.1	0	168	0	42
trout, rainbow, wild	3.5 oz.	5.8	1.6	0	149	0	56
whiting, fillet, bkd./brld., mixed species	3.5 oz.	1.7	0.4	0	115	0	131
Frozen (see also Fish/Shellfish Dinners and Entrees under FROZEN FOODS)							
Van de Kamp							
breaded fish fillet	1 fillet	9.5	1.5	9	140	0	135
breaded fish sticks	1 piece	2.8	0.4	4	48	0	65
Canned							
(NOTE: 2 oz. tuna ~ 1/4 cup serving)							
Bumble Bee							
salmon, pink	2.2 oz.	5.0	1.0	0	90	0	270
salmon, sockeye	2.2 oz.	7.0	2.0	0	110	0	270
tuna, chunk light in water	2 oz.	0.5	0.0	0	60	0	250
tuna, solid white in water	2 oz.	1.0	0.2	0	70	0	250
Chicken of the Sea							
salmon, pink	2 oz.	5.0	1.0	0	90	0	270
salmon, red	2 oz.	7.0	2.0	0	110	0	270
tuna, chunk light in water	2 oz.	0.5	0.0	0	60	0	250
tuna, solid white in water	2 oz.	1.0	0.1	0	70	0	250
Libby's							
pink salmon	2 oz.	4.5	0.9	0	81	0	243
pink salmon, w/o skin & bone	2 oz.	2.0	0.0	0	71	0	222
sockeye salmon, red	2 oz.	6.3	1.4	0	99	0	243
S & W							
chunk tuna, light, in water	2 oz.	0.1	0.0	0	70	0	230
minced clams	1/4 cup	0.0	0.0	1	20	0	360
smoked oysters	2 oz.	6.0	2.0	6	100	4	210
sockeye salmon, red	2 oz.	6.3	1.4	0	99	0	243
whole oysters	2 oz.	3.0	0.0	2	70	2	160
Starkist tuna, chunk white in water	2 oz.	1.0	0.2	0	60	0	250

	Serving	Total Fat (g)	Saturated Fat (g)	Total Carbohydrate (g)	Total Calories	Dietary Fiber	Sodium (mg)
Under Wood							
sardines, w/mustard sauce	2 oz.	6.4	1.6	1	96	1	439
sardines, w/tomato sauce	2 oz.	5.9	1.6	2	96	1	514

Breads/Loaf Breads, Variety Breads, Sandwich Buns, Rolls, English
Muffins, Bagels
Criterion for general selection: ≤ 1 gram fat per ounce (≤ 2 grams fat per standard 2-ounce serving); in general 1 slice ~ 1 ounce. Additional criterion: ≥ 2 grams fiber per 2-ounce serving.

Loaf Breads

	Serving	Total Fat (g)	Saturated Fat (g)	Total Carbohydrate (g)	Total Calories	Dietary Fiber	Sodium (mg)
USDA averages (most frequently consumed)							
cracked wheat	2 slices	2.0	0.5	25	130	3	269
egg, 5″ × 3″ × 1/2″ slice	1 slice	2.4	0.6	19	115	1	197
French, 4″ × 2 1/2″ × 1 3/4″ slice	1 slice	1.9	0.4	33	175	2	390
Italian, medium slice	2 slices	1.4	0.4	20	108	1	234
mixed grain	2 slices	2.0	0.4	24	130	3	253
multigrain, low calorie, high fiber	2 slices	1.1	0.2	20	93	6	235
oat bran	2 slices	2.6	0.4	24	142	3	244
potato	2 slices	1.9	0.4	26	139	1	280
protein	2 slices	0.9	0.1	17	93	1	208
pumpernickel	2 slices	1.6	0.2	25	130	3	349
rice bran	2 slices	2.5	0.4	23	131	3	238
rye	2 slices	2.1	0.4	31	166	4	422
sourdough & Vienna, 4″ × 2 1/2″ × 1 3/4″ slice	1 slice	1.9	0.4	33	175	2	390
sprouted wheat	2 slices	2.1	0.5	25	135	2	276
wheat & wheat berry	2 slices	2.1	0.5	24	130	2	265
white, enriched	2 slices	1.8	0.3	25	134	1	269
white, no salt added	2 slices	1.8	0.4	25	134	1	14
whole wheat	2 slices	2.4	0.5	26	138	4	295
Ener-G Foods, wheat-free breads							
harvest	1 slice	0.3	0.1	33	134	3	360
hi-fiber	1 slice	3.0	0.0	20	100	2	60
Natural Ovens							
better white	2 slices	2.0	0.0	38	160	4	150
cracked wheat	2 slices	2.0	0.0	32	160	6	140
health max	2 slices	2.0	0.0	32	160	6	160
hunger filler	2 slices	2.0	0.0	26	120	10	180

	Serving	Total Fat (g)	Saturated Fat (g)	Total Carbohydrate (g)	Total Calories	Dietary Fiber	Sodium (mg.)
mild rye	2 slices	1.0	0.0	26	140	8	140
multigrain	2 slices	2.0	0.0	28	140	6	180
nutty natural	2 slices	2.0	0.0	32	140	10	140
100% whole grain	2 slices	2.0	0.0	28	140	8	160
original lo-carb	2 slices	4.0	0.0	16	120	10	140
soft white	2 slices	2.0	0.0	30	140	6	140
sunny millet	2 slices	2.0	0.0	28	120	10	160
Pepperidge Farm							
cracked wheat, thin sliced	2 slices	2.0	0.0	24	140	1	280
French	2 slices	3.0	2.0	50	260	2	560
honey bran, old-fashioned	2 slices	2.0	0.0	34	180	4	320
Jewish rye, with or w/o seeds	2 slices	2.0	1.0	30	160	2	420
light seven grain	2 slices	0.7	0.0	19	93	3	213
light sourdough	2 slices	0.7	0.0	18	87	3	213
light Vienna	2 slices	0.7	0.3	19	87	3	200
light wheat	2 slices	0.7	0.3	19	87	3	193
nine grain	2 slices	2.0	0.0	32	180	4	340
oatmeal	2 slices	1.0	0.0	24	120	0	320
onion rye	2 slices	2.0	1.0	30	160	2	420
potato	2 slices	3.0	1.0	36	180	6	520
pumpernickel	2 slices	2.0	1.0	30	160	2	460
whole wheat, thin sliced	2 slices	2.0	0.0	22	120	1	240
Natural Whole Grain, breads w/100% whole wheat							
crunchy grains	1 slice	1.5	0.0	15	90	3	150
German dark wheat	1 slice	1.0	0.0	15	90	3	140
hearty bran	1 slice	1.5	0.0	15	90	3	130
honey oat	1 slice	1.5	0.0	15	90	2	135
multigrain	1 slice	2.0	0.0	15	90	3	150
nine grain	1 slice	1.0	0.0	15	90	3	140
oat bran	1 slice	1.5	0.0	15	90	2	115
seven grain	1 slice	2.0	0.0	18	100	2	180
whole wheat	1 slice	1.0	0.0	16	90	2	135
Variety Breads							
B & M brown raisin	2 slices	1.0	0.0	58	260	4	720
Natural Ovens							
Glorious	2 slices	1.0	0.0	30	140	4	140
Happiness	2 slices	2.0	0.0	30	140	6	140

	Serving	Total Fat (g)	Saturated Fat (g)	Total Carbohydrate (g)	Total Calories	Dietary Fiber	Sodium (mg)
Pepperidge Farm							
apple walnut swirl	1 slice	2.0	0.5	14	80	1	120
cinnamon	1 slice	2.5	0.5	14	80	2	115
fully baked French style	1 slice	1.5	0.5	24	120	1	260
raisin cinnamon swirl	1 slice	1.5	0.5	14	80	1	105
twin French or sourdough	1 slice	1.5	0.5	26	130	1	270
Sandwich Buns/Rolls/Pocket Breads							
Pepperidge Farm rolls							
club, brown 'n serve	1 roll	1.5	0.0	22	120	2	240
dinner, country style	1 roll	1.0	0.3	7	50	0	77
dinner, finger, w/poppy seeds	1 roll	1.5	0.5	7	50	0	77
dinner, Parker House	1 roll	1.5	0.5	7	50	0	77
frankfurter, Dijon	1 roll	3.0	1.5	23	140	2	240
French, brown 'n serve (2 pkg.)	1 roll	4.0	1.0	68	360	4	800
French, brown 'n serve (3 pkg.)	1 roll	2.5	0.5	45	240	3	490
French, seven grain	1 roll	2.0	0.0	19	80	2	270
English Muffins							
Pepperidge Farm							
cinnamon raisin	1 muffin	1.0	0.0	28	140	2	230
plain	1 muffin	1.0	0.0	26	253	2	250
seven grain	1 muffin	1.0	0.0	26	130	2	230
sourdough	1 muffin	1.0	0.0	26	130	2	250
Thomas							
honey wheat	1 muffin	0.5	0.0	27	130	2	180
oat bran	1 muffin	1.0	0.0	26	130	2	210
Bagels, fresh (USDA averages most frequently consumed)							
cinnamon raisin, 3 1/2"	1 bagel	1.2	0.2	39	195	2	229
cinnamon raisin, 4 1/2"	1 bagel	2.0	0.3	65	323	3	380
egg, 3 1/2"	1 bagel	1.5	0.3	37	198	2	359
egg, 4 1/2"	1 bagel	2.3	0.5	58	306	3	555
oat bran, 3 1/2"	1 bagel	0.9	0.1	38	181	2	360
onion, 3 1/2"	1 bagel	1.1	0.2	38	195	2	379
plain	1 bagel	1.1	0.2	38	195	2	379
poppy seed, 3 1/2"	1 bagel	1.1	0.2	38	195	2	379
sesame seed, 3 1/2"	1 bagel	1.1	0.2	38	195	2	379

	Serving	Total Fat (g)	Saturated Fat (g)	Total Carbohydrate (g)	Total Calories	Dietary Fiber (g)	Sodium (mg)

Breads/Refrigerated and Frozen Breads, Biscuits, Rolls
Criterion for general selection: ≤ 3 grams fat per 2-ounce serving
Refrigerated Breads, Biscuits, Rolls (dairy case)
Pillsbury

	Serving	Total Fat (g)	Saturated Fat (g)	Total Carbohydrate (g)	Total Calories	Dietary Fiber (g)	Sodium (mg)
bread sticks	1 piece	2.0	0.0	19	110	1	290
bread sticks, garlic & herb	1 piece	3.5	0.8	13	90	0	290
buttermilk	1 biscuit	1.4	0.3	30	154	0	547
country style	1 biscuit	0.7	0.0	10	50	0	180
French loaf	1/5 loaf	2.0	1.0	27	150	1	390
wheat loaf	1/4 loaf	2.0	0.5	7	50	1	150

Frozen Breads, Bagels, English Muffins, Rolls
Lender's

	Serving	Total Fat (g)	Saturated Fat (g)	Total Carbohydrate (g)	Total Calories	Dietary Fiber (g)	Sodium (mg)
blueberry, 4"	1 bagel	1.5	0.3	53	264	2	427
blueberry, big n' crusty,	1 bagel	0.8	0.2	46	214	2	406
blueberry, premium, 3"	1 bagel	1.3	0.3	43	209	2	409

Tortillas
Mission Foods

	Serving	Total Fat (g)	Saturated Fat (g)	Total Carbohydrate (g)	Total Calories	Dietary Fiber (g)	Sodium (mg)
flour, soft taco,	1 tortilla	3.1	0.4	25	146	0	249

Breads/Muffins, Pastries, Sweet Breakfast Breads, Bread Mixes
Criterion for general selection: ≤ 4 grams fat per 2-ounce serving
Bread Mixes
Arrowhead Mills bread mixes

	Serving	Total Fat (g)	Saturated Fat (g)	Total Carbohydrate (g)	Total Calories	Dietary Fiber (g)	Sodium (mg)
cornbread	1/2 cup	2.0	0.0	48	240	8	540
kamut	1/2 cup	1.5	0.0	47	212	8	288
multigrain	1/2 cup	1.5	0.0	47	242	5	288
rye	1/2 cup	0.8	0.0	50	242	5	288
white	1/2 cup	0.8	0.0	47	227	3	258
whole wheat	1/2 cup	1.5	0.0	47	227	8	288

Pillsbury

	Serving	Total Fat (g)	Saturated Fat (g)	Total Carbohydrate (g)	Total Calories	Dietary Fiber (g)	Sodium (mg)
banana	2 oz.	2.6	0.0	45	223	2	326
blueberry	2 oz.	2.4	0.0	46	220	1	252
bread, nut	2 oz.	5.5	0.8	43	236	2	284
cranberry	2 oz.	2.3	0.0	46	215	2	230
date	2 oz.	2.2	0.0	47	218	1	218
lemon poppy seed	2 oz.	6.9	1.5	41	245	1	230
pumpkin	2 oz.	2.6	0.0	45	223	1	326

Muffins (packaged, frozen, mixes)
Entenmann's

	Serving	Total Fat (g)	Saturated Fat (g)	Total Carbohydrate (g)	Total Calories	Dietary Fiber (g)	Sodium (mg)
blueberry	1 muffin	7.0	1.5	24	160	1	210

	Serving	Total Fat (g)	Saturated Fat (g)	Total Carbohydrate (g)	Total Calories	Dietary Fiber	Sodium (mg)
blueberry, fat- & cholesterol-free	1 muffin	0.0	0.0	26	120	1	220
General Mills, prepared from 2-oz. mix							
cornmeal	1 muffin	3.5	1.0	25	140	1	290
low-fat variety	1 muffin	1.4	0.1	48	216	0	397
Krusteaz							
apple cinnamon	1 muffin	4.5	1.5	33	180	1	330
apple cinnamon, low fat	1 muffin	1.4	0.3	47	213	1	516
basic, low fat	1 muffin	1.8	0.6	46	214	1	530
blueberry, frozen, prepared from 2 oz. mix	1 muffin	9.2	1.7	28	208	1	160
blueberry, low fat	1 muffin	1.0	0.0	29	130	1	300
oat bran, low fat	1 muffin	2.0	1.0	32	160	1	320
whole wheat, low fat	1 muffin	1.0	0.0	32	150	1	380
Martha White, mixes							
apple cinnamon	1/3 cup	3.5	1.0	30	162	1	343
apple cinnamon, low fat	1/3 cup	2.7	0.7	45	213	1	267
blueberry, low fat	1/3 cup	2.7	0.7	45	213	1	267
cornmeal, yellow	1/3 cup	3.5	1.0	31	162	1	283
lemon poppy seed	1/3 cup	5.3	1.3	35	200	1	307
strawberry, low fat	1/3 cup	2.7	0.7	45	213	1	267
Pepperidge Farm							
apple oatmeal	1 muffin	3.5	0.5	28	160	3	190
blueberry	1 muffin	2.5	0.0	27	140	2	190
cornmeal	1 muffin	3.0	0.0	27	150	1	190
raisin bran	1 muffin	2.5	0.5	30	150	4	260
Danish, Sweet Rolls, Coffee Cakes, Breakfast Pastries							
Entenmann's							
Buns, cinnamon raisin, fat- & cholesterol-free	1 each	0.0	0.0	36	160	1	125
Cakes, fat- & cholesterol-free							
blueberry crunch, fat- & cholesterol-free	1 piece	0.0	0.0	32	140	2	200
coffee, cinnamon apple	1 piece	0.0	0.0	29	130	2	110
marble loaf	1 piece	0.0	0.0	29	130	1	190
Pastries, fat- & cholesterol-free							
apricot	1 piece	0.0	0.0	34	150	1	110
cinnamon apple twist	1 piece	0.0	0.0	35	150	1	110

	Serving	Total Fat (g)	Saturated Fat (g)	Total Carbohydrate (g)	Total Calories	Dietary Fiber	Sodium (mg)
lemon twist	1 piece	0.0	0.0	31	130	1	140
raspberry cheese	1 piece	0.0	0.0	32	140	1	110

Pancakes, Waffles, French Toast (frozen and mixes)

Arrowhead Mills

	Serving	Total Fat (g)	Saturated Fat (g)	Total Carbohydrate (g)	Total Calories	Dietary Fiber	Sodium (mg)
pancake and waffles mixes							
blue corn	½ cup dry	3.0	0.0	43	227	5	197
buckwheat	½ cup dry	2.3	0.0	38	212	8	333
buttermilk	½ cup dry	1.5	0.0	52	250	3	1155
multigrain	½ cup dry	1.0	0.0	48	240	6	520
oat bran	½ cup dry	2.3	0.0	38	212	9	243
original	½ cup dry	0.9	0.2	51	236	2	1127
whole grain	½ cup dry	1.0	0.0	48	240	8	520
Aunt Jemima							
pancakes, frozen							
blueberry	3 pancakes	4.0	1.4	46	249	1	789
buttermilk	3 pancakes	3.7	0.9	45	240	1	778
original	3 pancakes	3.7	1.3	47	246	1	777
waffles, frozen							
apple cinnamon	1 waffle	2.8	0.7	14	88	1	252
blueberry	1 waffle	2.6	0.7	15	88	1	342
buttermilk	1 waffle	2.9	0.7	14	90	1	308
original	1 waffle	3.0	0.8	15	98	1	282
raisin	1 waffle	2.0		18	100	1	263
whole grain	1 waffle	1.4	0.4	15	77	2	338
pancakes, dry mix							
buckwheat	½ cup	1.7	0.3	47	206	7	1159
buttermilk, reduced calorie	½ cup	2.1	0.6	42	200	8	960
pancake & waffle, dry mix							
whole wheat	½ cup	1.2	0.2	52	237	5	1248
Eggo, frozen							
buttermilk pancakes	3 pancakes	8.0	1.5	44	270	1	610
waffles							
apple cinnamon	1 waffle	3.5	0.8	15	100	1	200
blueberry	1 waffle	3.5	0.8	15	100	1	205
buttermilk	1 waffle	3.5	0.8	14	95	1	210
golden oat	1 waffle	1.1	0.2	13	69	1	135
homestyle	1 waffle	3.5	0.8	15	95	1	220
homestyle, low fat	1 waffle	1.3	0.3	16	80	1	150

	Serving	Total Fat (g)	Saturated Fat (g)	Total Carbohydrate (g)	Total Calories	Dietary Fiber (g)	Sodium (mg)
Nutri-Grain, blueberry, low fat	1 waffle	1.0	0.1	15	73	1	207
Special K, fat-free	1 waffle	0.0	0.0	13	60	1	140
strawberry	1 waffle	3.5	0.8	15	100	1	210
Gold Medal							
buttermilk, complete, from dry mix	2 pancakes	5.0	0.0	36	200	0	600
Hungry Jack							
pancakes, dry mixes							
buttermilk, complete	1/2 cup	2.3	0.0	49	243	2	864
extra light, complete	1/2 cup	3.0	0.8	46	227	2	909
original	1/2 cup	2.3	0.0	49	227	1	970
potato	1/2 cup	0.0	0.0	64	280	4	1440
Krusteaz							
blueberry, frozen	3 pancakes	5.4	1.3	51	281	3	722
buckwheat, from dry mix	3 (5-in.)	5.0	1.0	63	340	6	1010
buttermilk, from dry mix	3 (5-in.)	4.0	1.0	56	300	3	1180
buttermilk, frozen	3 pancakes	4.0	1.1	37	211	2	545
whole wheat & honey, from dry mix	3 (5-in.)	2.5	0.5	58	300	4	640

Pasta/Noodles/Macaroni (including noodle mixes)—see also

FROZEN FOODS, Italian Dinners & Entrees

Criterion for general selection: ≤ 4 grams fat per serving (2 ounces dry or 1 cup cooked)

American Italian Pasta Company brands include Anthony's, Global A1, Golden Grain, Luxury, Mrs. Grass, Mueller's, Pennsylvania Dutch, Ronco. Nutritional values are the same for all enriched pastas in all these brands.

	Serving	Total Fat (g)	Saturated Fat (g)	Total Carbohydrate (g)	Total Calories	Dietary Fiber (g)	Sodium (mg)
bow ties, elbow, fettuccine, lasagna, linguine, shells, spaghetti, vermicelli	2 oz. dry	0.8	0.2	42	206	2	3
egg noodles	2 oz. dry	2.2	0.7	40	213	2	13
Di Giorno (fresh/dairy case)							
angel hair, fettuccine, liguine, plain,							
ravioli, cheese, light	2 oz.	3.9	2.3	22	157	1	225
spinach, herb	2 oz.	1.2	0.0	30	160	2	112
tortelloni, pepper, lemon chicken	2 oz.	3.1	1.9	26	166	1	179
tortelloni, portobello mushroom	2 oz.	3.7	2.7	25	164	2	260

	Serving	Total Fat (g)	Saturated Fat (g)	Total Carbohydrate (g)	Total Calories	Dietary Fiber (g)	Sodium (mg)
Ener-G Foods							
spaghetti, brown rice	2 oz. dry	0.5	0.0	43	211	1	
spaghetti, wheat free, low protein	2 oz. dry	0.1	0.0	48	194	0	
spaghetti, white rice, wheat-free	2 oz. dry	0.1	0.0	44	214	0	
Kraft Light Italian Pasta Salad	¾ cup	2.0	1.0	35	190	2	740

New World Pasta brands include Albadoro, American Beauty, Catelli, Creamette, Lancia, Monder, Prince, Ronzoni, San Giorgio, Skinner. Nutritional values are the same for all enriched pastas in all these brands.

	Serving	Total Fat (g)	Saturated Fat (g)	Total Carbohydrate (g)	Total Calories	Dietary Fiber (g)	Sodium (mg)
bow ties, elbow, fettuccine, lasagna, shells, spaghetti, vermicelli	2 oz. dry	0.8	0.2	42	206	2	3
egg noodles	2 oz. dry	2.2	0.7	40	213	2	13
Westbrae Natural							
angel hair, corn, dry	2 oz. dry	1.5	0.0	46	210	0	15
lasagna, spinach, organic	2 oz. dry	2.2	0.0	38	196	9	22
ramen, including buckwheat brown rice, & spinach	2 oz. dry	0.8	0.0	42	194	3	239
spaghetti noodles, whole wheat, organic	2 oz. dry	1.5	0.0	39	200	9	10
spaghetti, spinach, organic	2 oz. dry	2.0	0.0	38	180	8	20

Rice/Rice Mixes—see also FROZEN FOODS, Side Dishes
Criterion for general selection: ≤ 2 grams fat and ≥ 2 grams fiber per serving (2 oz. dry or 1 cup cooked)

	Serving	Total Fat (g)	Saturated Fat (g)	Total Carbohydrate (g)	Total Calories	Dietary Fiber (g)	Sodium (mg)
Arrowhead Mills rices, dry							
basmati, brown, long grain	2 oz.	1.3	0.0	43	197	3	0
brown, long grain	2 oz.	1.3	0.0	43	197	3	0
brown, medium grain	2 oz.	1.3	0.0	44	201	3	0
brown, quick, original	2 oz.	1.4	0.0	43	202	3	0
brown, short grain	2 oz.	1.3	0.0	47	224	3	0
Green Giant, frozen dishes							
pilaf, w/veg	1 pkg.	3.0	1.5	44	230	3	1020
w/veg medley	1 pkg.	3.0	1.5	46	240	3	880
white & wild, w/veg	1 pkg.	5.0	0.5	45	250	3	1000
La Choy							
La Choy fried rice (canned)	1 cup	1.1	0.2	54	241	2	1044

Serving	Total Fat (g)	Saturated Fat (g)	Total Carbohydrate (g)	Total Calories	Dietary Fiber	Sodium (mg)
Lundberg Family Foods, ¹/₄ cup dry = ³/₄ cup prepared according to package directions						
Gourmet Natural Brown Rices and Blends						
black japonica, field blend ¹/₄ cup dry	2.0	0.0	38	170	3	0
Christmas, brown ¹/₄ cup dry	1.5	0.0	37	170	3	0
country wild, blend ¹/₄ cup dry	1.5	0.0	35	150	3	0
jubilee, blend ¹/₄ cup dry	1.5	0.0	39	170	3	0
royal, aromatic ¹/₄ cup dry	2.0	0.0	38	170	2	0
wehani, aromatic ¹/₄ cup dry	1.5	0.0	38	170	3	0
wild blend ¹/₄ cup dry	1.5	0.0	35	150	3	0
Nutra-Farmed varieties from Lundberg						
California brown basmati ¹/₄ cup dry	2.0	0.0	38	170	2	0
long-grain brown ¹/₄ cup dry	2.0	0.0	37	170	3	0
short-grain brown ¹/₄ cup dry	1.5	0.0	40	170	3	0
One-Step Entrees, prepared						
chili 1 cup	1.0	0.0	42	180	5	420
curry 1 cup	1.0	0.0	38	160	5	400
garlic basil 1 cup	1.0	0.0	37	160	5	480
olde world pilaf 1 ¹/₂ cups	3.0	0.5	73	340	10	5
Organic Natural Brown Rices and Blends						
California basmati & wild blend ¹/₄ cup dry	1.5	0.0	34	150	2	0
wehani, aromatic ¹/₄ cup dry	1.5	0.0	38	170	3	0
wild ¹/₄ cup dry	0.5	0.0	34	160	3	0
wild blend ¹/₄ cup dry	1.5	0.0	35	150	3	0
Organic Quick Brown Rices, ¹/₂ package = 1 cup prepared according to directions						
exotic wild & mushroom ¹/₂ pkg.	3.0	1.0	53	260	4	800
hearty harvest quick brown ¹/₃ cup dry	1.0	0.0	30	140	3	15
picante Spanish fiesta ¹/₂ pkg.	2.5	0.5	53	260	5	670
roasted garlic pesto ¹/₂ pkg.	3.5	1.0	52	260	5	830
savory vegetarian chicken ¹/₂ pkg.	2.5	0.5	53	260	5	910
Minute rices, prepared according to package directions						
brown, instant 1 cup	2.3	0.0	51	257	3	15

	Serving	Total Fat (g)	Saturated Fat (g)	Total Carbohydrate (g)	Total Calories	Dietary Fiber (g)	Sodium (mg)
Rice-A-Roni rice dishes, dry, prepared according to package directions							
long grain & wild, w/chicken & almond flavor	2 oz.	2.1	0.3	41	195	2	893
red beans, w/rice	2 oz.	1.1	0.2	40	189	4	897
rice pilaf, long grain & wild	2 oz.	0.5	0.1	43	190	2	837
savory chicken vegetable flavor, low fat	2 oz.	1.1	0.2	40	193	2	771
Spanish	2 oz.	0.8	0.1	40	187	2	991
S & W, dry							
brown, long grain	2 oz.	1.4	0.0	43	202	2	0
brown, quick	2 oz.	1.3	0.0	43	197	3	7
wild	2 oz.	0.8	0.0	43	212	2	0
Uncle Ben's							
rice bowls							
barbeque flavor	1 bowl	4.5	1.5	85	430	4	1030
beef & broccoli, spicey	1 bowl	4.5	1.5	62	370	5	1550
chicken & vegetable	1 bowl	5.0	1.5	56	360	3	1020
chicken bombay	1 bowl	5.0	1.0	76	440	4	740
chicken, honey Dijon	1 bowl	3.5	0.5	73	400	3	740
chicken, sweet & sour	1 bowl	3.0	0.5	65	360	2	620
chicken, Szechuan	1 bowl	4.0	1.0	58	360	3	1800
chicken, teriyaki	1 bowl	3.5	0.5	66	380	3	1450
southwest-style black bean & vegetable	1 bowl	4.5	1.0	68	360	10	1250
teriyaki stir-fry vegetable	1 bowl	3.0	0.5	74	360	4	1360
rice pilafs, long grain & wild, dry							
harvest vegetable	2 oz.	0.7	0.1	41	185	2	763
seasoned, flavored & blended rices							
broccoli cheese flavor	2 oz.	1.9	1.1	42	200	2	758
Cajun	2 oz.	0.5	0.0	41	189	2	769
golden harvest	2 oz.	0.6	0.0	43	193	2	0
Mexican Fiesta flavor	2 oz.	0.7	0.4	42	193	2	705
whole-grain brown & wild, blend	2 oz.	1.5	0.5	41	199	2	589
unseasoned rices							

	Serving	Total Fat (g)	Saturated Fat (g)	Total Carbohydrate (g)	Total Calories	Dietary Fiber	Sodium (mg)
brown, long whole grain	2 oz.	1.8	0.0	42	192	2	0
wild, 100% pure	2 oz.	1.3	0.0	42	199	2	0

Beans and Peas, Canned

Criterion for general selection: ≤ 2 grams fat per ¹/₂ cup serving

	Serving	Total Fat (g)	Saturated Fat (g)	Total Carbohydrate (g)	Total Calories	Dietary Fiber	Sodium (mg)
B & M baked beans							
barbeque flavor	¹/₂ cup	1.0	0.0	33	170	6	460
99% fat-free, vegetarian	¹/₂ cup	1.0	0.0	31	170	7	220
red kidney	¹/₂ cup	2.0	0.5	32	170	6	440
with natural honey flavor	¹/₂ cup	1.5	0.0	30	170	8	450
yellow eye	¹/₂ cup	3.0	0.5	30	180	8	450
Bush's Best							
baked beans, barbeque flavor	¹/₂ cup	1.0	0.0	32	160	6	510
baked beans, Boston style	¹/₂ cup	1.5	0.0	32	170	6	440
baked beans, country style	¹/₂ cup	1.0	0.0	33	170	7	680
baked beans, homestyle	¹/₂ cup	1.5	0.0	28	150	8	480
baked beans, w/maple-cured bacon	¹/₂ cup	1.0	0.5	28	150	7	620
baked beans, onion	¹/₂ cup	1.5	0.0	26	150	6	500
baked beans, original	¹/₂ cup	1.0	0.0	29	150	7	550
baked beans, vegetarian	¹/₂ cup	0.0	0.0	24	130	6	550
black beans	¹/₂ cup	0.5	0.0	20	100	7	460
chili-style beans, hot	¹/₂ cup	1.0	0.5	20	120	6	480
chili-style beans, medium	¹/₂ cup	1.0	0.5	20	120	6	480
chili-style beans, mild	¹/₂ cup	1.0	0.5	20	120	6	480
Great Northern beans	¹/₂ cup	0.5	0.0	18	110	7	400
kidney beans, dark red	¹/₂ cup	1.0	0.0	21	130	7	260
pinto beans	¹/₂ cup	0.0	0.0	19	110	6	390
refried beans, fat-free	¹/₂ cup	0.0	0.0	24	130	7	490
Campbell's beans							
baked, barbequed	¹/₂ cup	2.5	0.5	29	170	6	460
barbequed, old fashioned	¹/₂ cup	2.5	0.5	29	170	6	460
pork & beans, in tomato sauce	¹/₂ cup	2.0	0.5	24	130	6	420
Eden Food's organic beans							
adzuki, w/o added salt, fat-free	¹/₂ cup	0.0	0.0	19	110	5	10
baked, w/sorghum & mustard, fat-free	¹/₂ cup	0.0	0.0	27	150	7	130

	Serving	Total Fat (g)	Saturated Fat (g)	Total Carbohydrate (g)	Total Calories	Dietary Fiber	Sodium (mg)
black, w/ginger & lemon, fat-free	1/2 cup	0.0	0.0	21	120	7	200
chickpea/garbanzo, w/o added salt, organic	1/2 cup	1.5	0.0	19	120	5	10
chili, w/beans, w/jalapeno & pepper, fat-free	1/2 cup	0.0	0.0	21	130	7	250
kidney, w/o added salt, free, organic	1/2 cup	0.0	0.0	18	100	10	15 fat-
navy, w/o added salt, organic	1/2 cup	0.5	0.0	20	110	7	15
pinto, spicy, w/jalapeno & red pepper, fat-free	1/2 cup	0.0	0.0	24	125	7	195
pinto, w/o added salt, fat-free	1/2 cup	0.0	0.0	18	100	6	15
soybeans, black, w/o added salt	1/2 cup	1.5	0.0	9	90	5	0
Green Giant beans							
black	1/2 cup	0.0	0.0	18	100	5	400
butter	1/2 cup	0.0	0.0	16	90	4	450
chickpea/garbanzo	1/2 cup	1.5	0.0	18	110	5	380
Great Northern	1/2 cup	0.5	0.0	18	100	6	290
kidney, dark red	1/2 cup	0.0	0.0	20	110	6	340
kidney, light red	1/2 cup	0.0	0.0	20	110	6	340
pinto	1/2 cup	0.5	0.0	20	110	5	280
pork & beans, w/tomato sauce	1/2 cup	1.0	0.0	23	120	4	490
red	1/2 cup	0.5	0.0	19	100	6	350
Health Valley							
chili, w/black beans, spicy, vegetarian, fat-free	1/2 cup	0.0	0.0	15	120	7	160
chili, w/3 beans, mild, vegetarian, fat-free	1/2 cup	0.0	0.0	15	120	7	160
Heirloom brand							
Jackson wonder	1/2 cup	0.0	0.0	19	100	5	135
runner, scarlet	1/2 cup	0.0	0.0	20	100	7	140
soldier, European	1/2 cup	0.0	0.0	16	90	5	140
trout	1/2 cup	0.0	0.0	18	100	6	140
Old El Paso beans							
black	1/2 cup	1.0	0.0	17	110	7	400

	Serving	Total Fat (g)	Saturated Fat (g)	Total Carbohydrate (g)	Total Calories	Dietary Fiber	Sodium (mg)
black, refried	1/2 cup	2.0	0.0	18	110	6	340
chickpea/garbanzo	1/2 cup	1.5	0.0	16	100	4	340
Mexican	1/2 cup	0.0	0.0	19	110	7	630
pinto	1/2 cup	0.5	0.0	19	100	7	420
refried	1/2 cup	0.5	0.0	17	100	6	570
refried, fat-free	1/2 cup	0.0	0.0	18	100	6	480
refried, spicy, fat-free	1/2 cup	0.0	0.0	18	100	6	720
refried, vegetarian	1/2 cup	1.0	0.0	17	100	6	490
refried, w/cheese	1/2 cup	3.5	1.5	18	130	6	500
refried, w/green chilies	1/2 cup	0.5	0.0	17	100	6	720
Ortega beans							
black, in sauce	1/2 cup	1.5	0.0	22	120	5	560
refried	1/2 cup	1.5	0.0	22	120	5	560
Progresso beans							
black	1/2 cup	1.0	0.0	17	110	7	400
cannellini	1/2 cup	0.5	0.0	18	100	5	270
chickpea/garbanzo	1/2 cup	1.5	0.0	18	110	5	380
fava/broad	1/2 cup	0.5	0.0	20	110	5	250
kidney, dark red	1/2 cup	0.0	0.0	20	110	6	340
kidney, red	1/2 cup	0.5	0.0	20	110	8	280
pinto	1/2 cup	1.0	0.0	18	110	7	250
Rosarita							
black, whole	1/2 cup	0.0	0.0	18	80	5	390
refried, no fat	1/2 cup	0.0	0.0	17	90	5	590
refried, original	1/2 cup	2.0	1.0	18	100	5	510
refried, spicy	1/2 cup	2.0	1.0	18	100	6	630
refried, vegetarian	1/2 cup	2.0	0.0	18	100	5	520
S & W beans							
baked, brick-oven style	1/2 cup	0.5	0.0	32	160	7	620
baked, honey mustard	1/2 cup	0.0	0.0	31	130	7	500
baked, maple sugar	1/2 cup	0.5	0.0	29	150	6	80
baked, sweet bacon	1/2 cup	1.5	0.5	31	140	6	530
barbequed, texas style	1/2 cup	1.5	0.5	25	140	8	640
black	1/2 cup	0.0	0.0	17	70	6	520
black, 50% less salt	1/2 cup	0.0	0.0	17	70	6	260
butter	1/2 cup	0.0	0.0	18	70	5	440
chili w/beans	1/2 cup	1.0	0.0	23	110	6	580
white, small	1/2 cup	0.5	0.0	19	80	6	440

	Serving	Total Fat (g)	Saturated Fat (g)	Total Carbohydrate (g)	Total Calories	Dietary Fiber (g)	Sodium (mg)
Sun Vista beans							
black	½ cup	1.0	0.0	20	70	7	630
chili, w/beans	½ cup	1.0	0.5	24	110	7	360
Great Northern	½ cup	0.0	0.0	17	70	6	490
pinto	½ cup	0.5	0.0	12	80	3	530
Westbrae Natural organic beans							
black	½ cup	0.0	0.0	19	100	5	140
chickpea/garbanzo	½ cup	2.0	0.0	18	110	5	140
chili, kidney pinto & black	½ cup	0.0	0.0	19	100	5	150
Great Northern	½ cup	0.0	0.0	19	100	6	140
kidney	½ cup	0.0	0.0	18	100	5	140
pinto	½ cup	0.0	0.0	19	100	7	140
red	½ cup	0.0	0.0	19	100	7	140
salad mix, kidney, pinto, & garbanzo	½ cup	0.5	0.0	19	100	5	150
soybeans	½ cup	7.0	1.0	11	150	3	140

Canned Entrees/Main Dishes

Criterion for general selection: ≤ 8 grams fat per serving (~1 cup)

Chili

	Serving	Total Fat (g)	Saturated Fat (g)	Total Carbohydrate (g)	Total Calories	Dietary Fiber (g)	Sodium (mg)
Amy's organic chili							
black bean	1 cup	2.0	0.0	31	200	15	680
medium chili w/vegetables	1 cup	6.0	0.5	29	190	8	590
medium or spicy chili	1 cup	6.0	0.5	26	190	7	590
Health Valley 99% fat-free chili							
black bean or 3 bean	1 cup	1.0	0.0	28	160	12	320
burrito or enchilada	1 cup	1.0	0.0	30	160	12	390
fajita flavor	1 cup	1.0	0.0	30	160	12	390
lentil	1 cup	1.0	0.0	28	160	11	390
mild or spicy	1 cup	1.0	0.0	30	160	11	390
turkey w/beans	1 cup	3.0	1.0	34	220	8	480
Hormel chili							
chunky w/bean	1 cup	7.0	3.0	34	270	7	1240
hot w/beans	1 cup	7.0	3.0	34	270	7	1220
less sodium w/beans	1 cup	7.0	3.0	34	270	7	910
turkey w/beans, 99% fat-free	1 cup	3.0	1.0	28	200	5	1200
vegetarian	1 cup	1.0	0.0	38	200	7	780
Stagg chili, 99% fat-free varieties							
Silverado beef	1 cup	3.0	1.0	33	230	6	880

	Serving	Total Fat (g)	Saturated Fat (g)	Total Carbohydrate (g)	Total Calories	Dietary Fiber	Sodium (mg)
turkey ranchero	1 cup	3.0	1.0	31	240	6	880
vegetable garden	1 cup	1.0	0.0	37	200	7	870
Lunch Entrees (shelf-stable microwaveable meals)							
Armour Lunch Buckets							
lasagna	1 each	4.0	2.0	38	220	2	870
pasta 'n chicken	1 each	6.0	2.0	22	180	2	860
spaghetti 'n meatsauce	1 each	5.0	2.5	39	240	2	870
Chef Boyardee Microwave Main Meals							
beef ravioli suprema	1 each	4.0	2.0	52	290	5	1390
beans & pasta	1 each	1.0	0.2	44	200	10	1030
cheese ravioli suprema	1 each	4.0	2.0	52	290	5	1360
lasagna	1 each	8.0	3.5	41	290	5	1000
meat tortellini	1 each	4.0	1.5	53	220	6	980
noodles w/chicken	1 each	1.0	0.5	27	170	3	1120
spaghetti suprema	1 each	7.0	3.0	37	200	7	1000
zesty macaroni	1 each	8.0	3.0	40	290	5	1300
ziti in sauce	1 each	<1.0	0.0	52	210	7	1030
Dinty Moore							
chicken & dumplings	1 each	5.0	2.0	17	220	0	680
chicken w/gravy & mashed potatoes	1 each	4.0	1.5	24	220	2	1180
chicken w/noodles, micro meal	1 each	8.0	3.0	26	260	2	1150
roast beef w/gravy & mashed potatoes	1 each	5.0	2.0	25	240	2	860
Homestyle Express							
beef steak	1 bowl	7.0	1.5	52	330	2	1200
chicken salsa	1 bowl	5.0	1.0	47	310	2	760
four-cheese tortellini	1 bowl	4.5	1.0	34	190	4	1110
Hormel Kids' Kitchen							
Beefy Mac	1 each	5.0	2.5	24	180	2	820
mini ravioli	1 each	7.0	2.0	35	240	3	920
noodle rings & chicken	1 each	4.0	1.5	18	140	1	950
spaghetti rings & meatballs	1 each	7.0	2.0	35	250	3	1200
Hormel Micro Cup Meals							
macaroni & beef w/vegetables	1 each	8.0	3.0	37	285	6	920
spaghetti & meat sauce	1 each	5.0	2.0	33	220	4	670

	Serving	Total Fat (g)	Saturated Fat (g)	Total Carbohydrate (g)	Total Calories	Dietary Fiber	Sodium (mg)
Hormel Pasta Cups							
garden salsa	1 each	0.5	0.0	23	120	2	650
Mediterrean style	1 each	8.0	2.5	24	200	2	710
Hormel Rice Cups							
southwest style	1 each	3.5	1.0	25	150	2	1140
sweet & sour	1 each	1.0	0.0	37	190	2	710
teriyaki	1 each	1.5	0.0	35	190	2	1370
Pasta/Italian Dishes (Canned)							
Chef Boyardee							
ABC's/123's	1 cup	0.5	0.0	43	200	2	900
Beefaroni in tomato sauce	1 cup	2.9	1.2	31	185	3	800
beef ravioli in tomato & meat sauce	1 cup	5.4	2.5	37	230	4	1175
mini beef ravioli in tomato sauce	1 cup	4.7	1.8	41	240	3	1200
Franco-American							
ravioli w/pasta in tomato & cheese sauce	1 cup	3.5	1.5	42	230	2	1020
SpaghettiOs meatballs	1 cup	8.0	3.5	32	240	3	990
SpaghettiOs original	1 cup	1.0	0.5	37	180	3	890

Soups, Canned and Mixes

Criterion for general selection: ≤ 3 grams fat per 1-cup serving

	Serving	Total Fat (g)	Saturated Fat (g)	Total Carbohydrate (g)	Total Calories	Dietary Fiber	Sodium (mg)
Amy's Kitchen organic soups, ready to serve							
black bean & vegetable, low fat	1 cup	1.0	0.0	22	110	5	580
chicken noodle, vegetarian	1 cup	3.0	0.0	12	90	2	480
cream of tomato	1 cup	2.0	1.5	17	100	4	690
lentil	1 cup	4.0	0.5	19	130	9	590
lentil vegetable	1 cup	4.0	0.5	23	150	9	680
minestrone, low fat	1 cup	1.5	0.0	17	90	3	540
split pea, fat-free	1 cup	0.0	0.0	19	100	4	570
tomato bisque, chunky	1 cup	3.5	2.0	21	120	2	680
vegetable barley, low fat	1 cup	1.0	0.0	10	50	2	580
vegetable bouillon/broth, fat-free	1 cup	0.0	0.0	8	35	1	680
Campbell's canned condensed soups, reconstituted w/water							
beef consommé	1 cup	0.0	0.0	1	20	0	810
beef noodle	1 cup	2.5	0.5	9	70	<1	870

	Serving	Total Fat (g)	Saturated Fat (g)	Total Carbohydrate (g)	Total Calories	Dietary Fiber	Sodium (mg)
beef w/vegetables and barley	1 cup	1.5	1.0	15	90	3	890
beefy mushroom	1 cup	2.0	1.0	6	50	0	890
black bean	1 cup	2.0	0.0	19	110	5	900
California-style vegetable	1 cup	0.5	0.0	13	70	2	810
chicken alphabet	1 cup	2.0	1.0	12	80	1	880
chicken and dumplings	1 cup	3.0	1.0	10	80	1	960
chicken and stars	1 cup	2.0	0.5	12	80	1	940
chicken gumbo	1 cup	1.0	0.5	10	60	1	870
chicken noodle	1 cup	1.5	0.5	8	60	<1	890
chicken vegetable	1 cup	1.0	0.5	15	80	2	890
chicken w/rice	1 cup	1.5	0.5	14	80	1	820
chicken won ton	1 cup	1.0	0.5	6	45	0	870
cream of broccoli, 98% fat-free	1 cup	1.0	0.5	12	60	2	700
cream of celery, 98% fat-free	1 cup	3.0	1.0	8	60	1	780
cream of chicken, 98% fat-free	1 cup	2.0	1.0	10	70	1	890
cream of mushroom, 98% fat-free	1 cup	3.0	1.0	9	70	1	900
double noodle in chicken broth	1 cup	2.0	0.5	17	90	2	830
French onion	1 cup	1.5	0.5	6	45	1	900
fun shapes	1 cup	1.5	0.5	12	80	2	780
goldfish pasta in tomato soup	1 cup	0.5	0.0	28	130	1	720
goldfish pasta w/chicken in chicken broth	1 cup	1.5	0.5	11	70	1	800
green pea	1 cup	3.0	1.0	28	180	4	870
hearty vegetable w/pasta	1 cup	0.5	0.0	19	90	2	890
homestyle chicken noodle	1 cup	2.0	1.0	8	70	1	940
Manhattan clam chowder	1 cup	0.5	0.5	12	70	2	880
mega noodle in chicken broth	1 cup	1.5	0.5	13	80	0	800
minestrone	1 cup	1.0	0.5	17	90	3	960
New England clam chowder	1 cup	2.5	0.5	13	90	1	880
New England clam	1 cup	2.0	0.5	13	80	1	940

	Serving	Total Fat (g)	Saturated Fat (g)	Total Carbohydrate (g)	Total Calories	Dietary Fiber	Sodium (mg)
chowder, 98% fat-free							
old-fashioned tomato rice	1 cup	2.0	0.5	23	110	1	770
old-fashioned vegetable	1 cup	1.5	0.5	14	80	2	940
Scotch broth	1 cup	2.0	1.0	9	70	2	880
southwest-style chicken vegetable	1 cup	1.0	0.5	21	110	4	830
tomato	1 cup	0.0	0.0	20	90	1	710
tomato noodle	1 cup	0.5	0.0	25	120	2	660
turkey noodle	1 cup	2.0	1.0	9	70	1	890
vegetable	1 cup	0.5	0.5	20	100	3	890
vegetable beef	1 cup	1.0	0.5	15	80	3	890
vegetarian vegetable	1 cup	0.5	0.0	18	90	2	790
Campbell's chunky soups							
beef with country vegetables	1 cup	3.0	1.5	22	160	4	910
beef with white and wild rice	1 cup	2.5	1.5	24	150	2	960
classic chicken noodle	1 cup	2.5	1.0	16	100	2	860
grilled chicken w/vegetables and pasta	1 cup	1.5	0.5	15	110	2	890
grilled sirloin steak w/hearty vegetables	1 cup	2.0	1.0	19	130	4	920
hearty bean 'n' ham	1 cup	2.0	1.0	30	180	8	800
hearty chicken w/vegetables	1 cup	1.5	0.5	14	100	2	790
hearty vegetables w/pasta	1 cup	2.0	0.0	23	130	3	930
herb-roasted chicken w/potatoes and garlic	1 cup	1.5	1.0	17	110	3	870
honey-roasted ham w/potatoes	1 cup	2.5	1.0	20	130	3	810
old-fashioned vegetable beef	1 cup	2.5	1.5	18	130	6	910
pepper steak	1 cup	1.5	1.0	18	120	3	740
savory chicken w/white and wild rice	1 cup	1.5	0.5	19	120	2	840
seasoned rib roast w/potatoes and herbs	1 cup	1.0	1.0	17	110	3	890
slow-roasted beef w/mushrooms	1 cup	1.5	1.0	18	120	3	830
split pea 'n' ham	1 cup	2.5	1.0	27	170	4	780

	Serving	Total Fat (g)	Saturated Fat (g)	Total Carbohydrate (g)	Total Calories	Dietary Fiber	Sodium (mg)
steak 'n' potato	1 cup	2.0	0.5	18	130	2	920
Campbell's chunky microwavable bowls							
classic chicken noodle	1 cup	2.0	1.0	15	110	1	860
grilled chicken with pasta	1 cup	2.0	1.0	13	100	5	850
sirloin steak w/hearty vegetables	1 cup	2.0	0.5	18	130	3	920
Campbell's Healthy Request soups, reconstituted w/water							
chicken noodle	1 cup	2.0	1.0	8	60	1	450
chicken rice	1 cup	2.0	1.0	13	80	1	420
cream of celery	1 cup	2.0	1.0	11	70	0	430
cream of chicken	1 cup	2.5	1.0	12	70	1	450
cream of mushroom	1 cup	2.5	1.0	10	70	1	460
hearty chicken w/white and wild rice	1 cup	2.0	1.0	17	110	2	360
minestrone	1 cup	0.5	0.0	15	80	3	460
tomato	1 cup	1.5	0.5	18	90	1	450
vegetable	1 cup	1.0	0.0	20	100	3	480
vegetable beef	1 cup	1.0	0.5	15	90	3	480
Campbell's Kitchen Classics							
chicken noodle	1 cup	1.0	0.5	13	90	1	870
chicken w/white & wild rice	1 cup	1.0	0.5	18	100	2	800
lentil	1 cup	0.5	0.5	23	120	5	750
minestrone	1 cup	0.5	0.5	22	110	3	840
tomato	1 cup	0.0	0.0	24	100	3	760
vegetable	1 cup	0.5	0.0	22	100	3	820
Campbell's low-sodium soups							
chicken broth	1 can	0.5	0.5	1	25	0	140
Campbell's Select microwavable bowls							
beef w/portobello mushrooms and rice	1 cup	1.5	1.0	13	100	1	860
chicken w/egg noodles	1 cup	1.5	0.5	11	90	1	990
Italian-style wedding soup	1 cup	2.5	2.0	15	115	5	850
New England clam chowder, 98% fat-free	1 cup	1.5	0.5	15	110	3	890
Campbell's Select soups							
bean and ham	1 cup	1.0	0.5	30	170	7	680

	Serving	Total Fat (g)	Saturated Fat (g)	Total Carbohydrate (g)	Total Calories	Dietary Fiber	Sodium (mg)
beef w/portobello mushrooms and rice	1 cup	1.5	1.0	15	110	1	860
beef with roasted barley	1 cup	1.5	1.0	24	150	3	860
chicken & pasta w/roasted garlic	1 cup	1.5	0.5	16	110	2	840
chicken rice	1 cup	1.0	0.5	17	100	2	990
chicken vegetable	1 cup	0.5	0.0	18	100	3	830
chicken with egg noodles	1 cup	1.5	0.5	14	100	1	990
fiesta vegetable	1 cup	0.5	0.0	24	120	4	760
grilled chicken w/sun-dried tomatoes & mushrooms	1 cup	1.0	0.5	17	110	2	780
herbed chicken w/roasted vegetables	1 cup	0.5	0.5	14	90	1	890
honey-roasted chicken w/golden potatoes	1 cup	1.0	1.0	16	100	1	860
Italian-style wedding soup	1 cup	2.5	2.0	16	120	2	850
minestrone	1 cup	0.0	0.0	20	100	4	790
New England clam chowder, 98% fat-free	1 cup	1.5	0.5	19	110	2	860
roasted chicken w/long-grain rice & wild rice	1 cup	0.5	0.0	17	100	2	870
roasted chicken w/rotini & penne pasta	1 cup	1.0	0.5	16	100	2	860
rosemary chicken w/roasted potatoes	1 cup	0.5	0.0	18	100	2	880
savory lentil	1 cup	0.5	0.5	27	140	6	860
split pea w/ham	1 cup	1.0	0.5	29	160	5	860
tomato garden	1 cup	0.5	0.5	21	100	3	700
vegetable	1 cup	0.5	0.0	21	100	3	900
vegetable beef	1 cup	2.0	1.0	16	110	3	910
Campbell's Soup-at-Hand							
blended vegetable medley	1 container	2.0	1.5	21	110	3	970
chicken & stars	1 container	0.5	0.5	11	60	1	960
chicken with mini noodles	1 container	1.5	0.5	12	80	2	980
classic tomato	1 container	0.0	0.0	27	120	2	970
Mexican-style fiesta	1 container	3.0	1.0	22	130	3	930
pizza	1 container	0.5	0.5	17	130	2	850
Healthy Choice							
beef & ham	1 cup	2.5	1.0	29	170	6	480

	Serving	Total Fat (g)	Saturated Fat (g)	Total Carbohydrate (g)	Total Calories	Dietary Fiber	Sodium (mg)
beef & potato	1 cup	1.0	0.0	19	110	2	480
chicken corn chowder	1 cup	2.0	1.0	26	140	3	480
chicken & dumplings	1 cup	2.0	0.5	22	130	7	480
chicken & pasta	1 cup	2.0	0.5	18	110	2	480
chicken & rice	1 cup	3.0	1.0	12	90	2	480
chicken fiesta	1 cup	2.0	0.5	17	100	3	480
chicken w/roasted garlic	1 cup	2.0	0.5	19	120	2	480
chili beef	1 cup	2.0	1.0	31	170	8	480
clam chowder	1 cup	1.5	1.0	21	110	3	480
country vegetable	1 cup	0.5	0.0	22	100	4	480
creamy tomato	1 cup	1.5	1.0	22	100	2	480
garden vegetable	1 cup	1.0	0.0	25	120	4	480
hearty chicken	1 cup	2.0	0.5	22	120	3	480
Italian bean & pasta	1 cup	1.5	0.5	18	100	3	480
old-fashioned chicken noodle	1 cup	2.0	0.5	16	110	3	480
roasted Italian-style chicken	1 cup	2.0	1.0	18	120	4	480
split pea with ham	1 cup	2.5	1.0	30	170	4	480
turkey with rice	1 cup	1.5	0.0	16	90	3	480
vegetable beef	1 cup	1.0	0.0	24	130	4	480
vegetable clam chowder	1 cup	1.0	0.0	16	80	3	480
zesty gumbo	1 cup	2.0	1.0	16	100	3	480
Health Valley							
fat-free black bean & vegetable	1 cup	0.0	0.0	24	110	9	280
fat-free corn and vegetable	1 cup	0.0	0.0	17	70	7	135
fat-free 5-bean vegetable	1 cup	0.0	0.0	32	140	10	250
fat-free 14-garden vegetable	1 cup	0.0	0.0	17	80	4	250
fat-free Italian minestrone	1 cup	0.0	0.0	21	90	8	210
fat-free lentil & carrots	1 cup	0.0	0.0	25	100	4	220
fat-free pasta cacciatore	1 cup	0.0	0.0	20	100	4	290
fat-free pasta fagioli	1 cup	0.0	0.0	25	120	4	290
fat-free pasta Romano	1 cup	0.0	0.0	20	100	4	290
fat-free rotini & vegetables	1 cup	0.0	0.0	20	100	4	290
fat-free split pea & carrots	1 cup	0.0	0.0	17	110	4	230
fat-free super broccoli carotene	1 cup	0.0	0.0	16	70	7	240
fat-free tomato vegetable	1 cup	0.0	0.0	17	80	5	240
fat-free vegetable barley	1 cup	0.0	0.0	19	90	4	210

	Serving	Total Fat (g)	Saturated Fat (g)	Total Carbohydrate (g)	Total Calories	Dietary Fiber	Sodium (mg)
99% fat-free chicken noodle	1 cup	2.0	0.0	20	130	2	390
rich & hearty chicken noodle soup	1 cup	2.5	1.0	13	100	2	580
Health Valley dry soup mix cups, prepared according to package directions							
fat-free chicken-flavored noodles w/vegetable	1 cup	0.0	0.0	24	110	3	270
fat-free corn chowder with tomatoes	1 cup	0.0	0.0	21	100	3	270
fat-free creamy potato with broccoli	1 cup	0.0	0.0	17	80	3	290
fat-free garden split pea with carrots	1 cup	0.0	0.0	22	110	2	270
fat-free lentil with couscous	1 cup	0.0	0.0	28	130	5	270
fat-free pasta Italiano	1 cup	0.0	0.0	31	140	3	270
fat-free spicy black bean w/couscous	1 cup	0.0	0.0	29	130	5	290
fat-free zesty black bean w/rice	1 cup	0.0	0.0	22	100	4	240
Health Valley no-salt-added organic soups							
black bean	1 cup	1.0	0.0	25	130	5	25
lentil	1 cup	1.0	0.0	21	100	8	25
minestrone	1 cup	0.0	0.0	17	70	3	45
mushroom barley	1 cup	0.0	0.0	17	70	3	25
potato leek	1 cup	0.0	0.0	15	70	3	35
split pea	1 cup	0.0	0.0	23	110	8	115
tomato	1 cup	0.0	0.0	18	80	1	35
vegetable	1 cup	0.0	0.0	18	80	4	40
Health Valley organic soups							
black bean	1 cup	1.0	0.0	25	130	5	380
lentil	1 cup	1.0	0.0	21	100	8	380
minestrone	1 cup	0.0	0.0	17	110	3	380
mushroom barley	1 cup	0.0	0.0	17	70	3	380
potato leek	1 cup	0.0	0.0	15	70	3	230
split pea	1 cup	0.0	0.0	23	110	8	160
tomato	1 cup	0.0	0.0	18	80	1	380
vegetable	1 cup	0.0	0.0	18	80	4	380
Imagine organic natural soups							
creamy broccoli	1 cup	1.5	0.0	10	70	2	370
creamy butternut squash	1 cup	2.0	0.5	23	120	2	370

	Serving	Total Fat (g)	Saturated Fat (g)	Total Carbohydrate (g)	Total Calories	Dietary Fiber	Sodium (mg)
creamy portobella mushroom	1 cup	3.0	0.0	10	80	2	310
creamy potato leek	1 cup	2.5	0.0	14	90	2	380
creamy sweet corn	1 cup	3.0	0.0	15	100	1	340
creamy tomato	1 cup	1.5	0.0	17	90	1	520
free-range chicken broth	1 cup	0.5	0.0	2	20	<1	570
no-chicken broth	1 cup	0.5	0.0	4	20	<1	460
vegetable broth	1 cup	0.5	0.0	5	30	1	480
Knorr naturals, hearty soup mixes							
chunky potato w/roasted onion	1 cup	1.0	0.0	20	100	1	850
homestyle chicken-flavor noodle	1 cup	1.5	0.5	13	80	1	860
roasted vegetable w/long grain rice	1 cup	1.0	0.5	17	90	1	830
Knorr Savory soup mixes							
chicken flavor noodle	1 cup	1.5	1.0	11	70	1	650
cream of chicken and rice	1 cup	2.5	1.5	14	90	0	860
Mediterranean-style minestrone	1 cup	5.0	1.0	18	100	3	810
Knorr soup mixes, prepared							
cream of broccoli	1 cup	2.5	0.5	10	70	1	730
cream of spinach	1 cup	2.5	0.5	10	70	<1	760
French onion	1 cup	1.0	0.5	6	35	0	790
hot and sour	1 cup	1.5	0.5	8	45	0	880
leek	1 cup	2.5	1.0	10	70	0	850
roasted garlic herb	1 cup	1.5	0.5	13	80	0	860
spring vegetable	1 cup	0.0	0.0	5	25	1	610
tomato with basil	1 cup	2.5	1.0	13	80	0	920
vegetable	1 cup	1.5	0.5	10	60	2	880
Progresso, ready to serve							
beef barley	1 cup	1.9	0.7	20	142	3	470
beef barley, 99% fat-free	1 cup	1.6	0.7	17	137	4	528
beef vegetable	1 cup	1.5	0.6	25	154	6	405
chicken noodle	1 cup	1.6	0.4	9	76	1	460
chicken rice w/vegetable	1 cup	1.5	0.4	13	88	1	459
lentil	1 cup	1.5	0.3	20	126	6	443
minestrone	1 cup	2.5	0.4	20	123	1	470
split pea	1 cup	2.3	0.8	30	180	5	420

	Serving	Total Fat (g)	Saturated Fat (g)	Total Carbohydrate (g)	Total Calories	Dietary Fiber	Sodium (mg)
vegetable	1 cup	1.3	0.3	13	81	4	528
Westbrae Natural, vegetarian, ready to eat							
Alabama black bean gumbo	1 cup	0.0	0.0	26	140	6	530
Great Plains savory bean	1 cup	0.0	0.0	23	120	7	540
hearty Milano minestrone	1 cup	0.0	0.0	24	120	6	570
Louisiana bean stew	1 cup	0.0	0.0	25	130	7	550
Mediterranean lentil	1 cup	0.0	0.0	24	140	10	540
New York unchicken noodle	1 cup	1.0	0.0	10	60	4	820
old-world split pea	1 cup	0.0	0.0	28	150	6	590
Santa Fe vegetable	1 cup	0.0	0.0	31	160	8	380
spicy southwest vegetable	1 cup	0.0	0.0	25	130	6	540
Westbrae Natural, semi-condensed, prepared according to package directions							
California unchicken broth	1 cup	0.5	0.0	2	15	0	890
Monte Carlo creamy mushroom	1 cup	3.0	1.5	10	70	0	680
Tuscany tomato	1 cup	0.0	0.0	16	70	0	710

Sauces and Gravies, Canned, Jars, and Mixes

Criterion for general selection: ≤ 4 grams fat per ¹/₂ cup serving (or ≤ 2 grams fat per ¹/₄ cup serving)

Pasta and Pizza sauces

	Serving	Total Fat (g)	Saturated Fat (g)	Total Carbohydrate (g)	Total Calories	Dietary Fiber	Sodium (mg)
Amy's Kitchen organic sauces							
family marinara	¹/₂ cup	1.0	0.0	8	50	3	590
garlic mushroom	¹/₂ cup	7.0	2.5	10	120	3	680
marinara, low sodium	¹/₂ cup	1.0	0.0	7	40	1	100
pomodoro zucca	¹/₂ cup	0.5	0.0	6	30	1	590
puttanesca	¹/₂ cup	2.0	0.0	5	40	1	680
tomato basil	¹/₂ cup	6.0	1.0	11	110	3	580
wild mushroom	¹/₂ cup	2.5	0.0	7	60	2	580
Classico pasta sauces							
cabernet marinara w/herbs	¹/₂ cup	2.0	0.0	10	60	2	400
fire-roasted tomato & garlic	¹/₂ cup	0.5	0.0	10	50	2	320
garden vegetable primavera	¹/₂ cup	1.0	0.0	11	60	2	610
Italian sausage with peppers & onions	¹/₂ cup	2.0	1.0	13	90	2	470
mushrooms & ripe olives	¹/₂ cup	1.0	0.5	11	60	2	390
roasted chicken with parmesan & garlic	¹/₂ cup	2.0	0.5	13	90	2	470
roasted garlic	¹/₂ cup	1.0	0.0	11	60	2	220

	Serving	Total Fat (g)	Saturated Fat (g)	Total Carbohydrate (g)	Total Calories	Dietary Fiber	Sodium (mg)
spicy red pepper	¹/₂ cup	1.5	0.0	7	60	2	300
spicy tomato & pesto	¹/₂ cup	4.0	0.0	11	90	2	470
sundried tomato	¹/₂ cup	3.0	1.0	11	80	2	390
sweet basil marinara	¹/₂ cup	1.0	0.0	13	70	1	280
tomato & basil	¹/₂ cup	1.0	0.0	11	60	2	310
triple mushroom	¹/₂ cup	2.0	0.5	12	80	3	390
Contadina sauces							
marinara, deluxe	¹/₂ cup	3.5	0.6	9	73	2	469
pizza, deluxe	¹/₂ cup	1.5	0.6	11	68	3	233
pizza, original	¹/₂ cup	0.0	0.0	12	60	2	680
pizza, w/four cheeses	¹/₂ cup	1.0	0.0	12	60	2	780
pizza, w/pepperoni flavor	¹/₂ cup	2.0	0.0	10	70	1	780
spaghetti	¹/₂ cup	1.6	0.2	12	70	2	563
Del Monte sauces (canned)							
spaghetti, four cheese	¹/₂ cup	2.0	0.0	15	70	3	680
spaghetti, garlic & herb, chunky	¹/₂ cup	2.0	0.0	11	60	1	490
spaghetti, Italian herb, chunky	¹/₂ cup	1.0	0.0	12	60	1	520
spaghetti, tomato & basil	¹/₂ cup	1.0	0.0	16	70	3	600
spaghetti, traditional	¹/₂ cup	1.0	0.0	15	60	3	590
spaghetti, w/garlic & onion	¹/₂ cup	1.0	0.0	16	80	2	490
spaghetti, w/green peppers & mushrooms	¹/₂ cup	1.0	0.0	16	80	3	490
spaghetti, w/meat	¹/₂ cup	1.0	0.0	14	60	3	720
spaghetti, w/mushrooms	¹/₂ cup	1.0	0.0	14	60	2	630
Healthy Choice sauces							
pasta, garlic & herb	¹/₂ cup	0.0	0.0	13	60	3	320
pasta, garlic & mushroom	¹/₂ cup	0.0	0.0	10	45	2	390
pasta, garlic & onion	¹/₂ cup	0.0	0.0	9	40	2	390
pasta, Italian-style vegetables	¹/₂ cup	0.0	0.0	9	40	2	390
pasta, marinara w/burgundy wine	¹/₂ cup	0.5	0.0	11	50	2	370
pasta, mushroom, super chunky	¹/₂ cup	0.0	0.0	9	40	2	390
pasta, mushroom & sweet pepper, chunky	¹/₂ cup	0.0	0.0	9	45	2	390

	Serving	Total Fat (g)	Saturated Fat (g)	Total Carbohydrate (g)	Total Calories	Dietary Fiber	Sodium (mg)
pasta, roasted garlic & romano	½ cup	1.0	0.0	11	60	3	390
Heinz							
pizza, traditional, 100% natural, Prince	½ cup	0.5	0.1	10	54	3	592
Hunt's Angela Mia sauces (canned)							
marinara	½ cup	1.0	0.0	9	50	2	480
pizza, extra heavy	½ cup	0.0	0.0	10	50	4	420
pizza, fully prep	½ cup	0.0	0.0	10	40	2	500
Newman's Own sauces							
five cheese	½ cup	3.0	1.5	14	90	3	510
Fra Diavolo	½ cup	3.0	0.0	10	70	3	510
marinara	½ cup	2.0	0.0	9	60	3	590
mushroom marinara	½ cup	2.0	0.0	9	60	3	590
roasted garlic & peppers	½ cup	2.5	0.0	11	70	4	460
tomato & basil	½ cup	4.0	0.5	15	100	5	590
tomato & roasted garlic	½ cup	2.5	0.0	11	70	1	580
tomato peppers & spices	½ cup	2.0	0.0	9	60	3	590
Prego sauces							
diced onion & garlic	½ cup	3.0	0.5	19	110	3	420
extra chunky, garden combination	½ cup	1.0	0.5	16	90	3	480
extra chunky, garlic & cheese	½ cup	2.0	0.5	22	120	5	570
extra chunky, garlic supreme	½ cup	3.0	0.5	23	130	3	570
extra chunky, mushroom & diced onion	½ cup	3.0	1.0	18	110	3	500
extra chunky, mushroom & diced tomato	½ cup	3.0	1.0	19	110	3	510
extra chunky, mushroom & green pepper	½ cup	4.5	0.5	18	120	6	430
extra chunky, mushroom supreme	½ cup	4.5	0.5	21	130	3	490
extra chunky, mushroom w/spice	½ cup	4.0	0.0	19	120	3	510
extra chunky, tomato onion garlic	½ cup	3.5	1.0	19	110	3	480

	Serving	Total Fat (g)	Saturated Fat (g)	Total Carbohydrate (g)	Total Calories	Dietary Fiber	Sodium (mg)
extra chunky, tomato supreme	1/2 cup	3.0	0.5	20	120	3	580
extra chunky, vegetable supreme	1/2 cup	3.0	0.5	15	90	3	490
extra chunky, zesty basil	1/2 cup	1.5	0.5	22	110	3	510
extra chunky, zesty oregano	1/2 cup	3.0	0.5	25	130	3	540
marinara	1/2 cup	6.0	1.5	12	110	3	670
mushroom Parmesan	1/2 cup	3.5	1.0	19	120	3	570
three cheese	1/2 cup	2.0	1.0	18	100	3	460
tomato & basil	1/2 cup	3.0	0.5	19	110	3	420
tomato Parmesan	1/2 cup	3.0	1.0	19	120	3	570
traditional, 100% natural	1/2 cup	5.1	1.1	21	137	4	559
w/mushrooms	1/2 cup	5.0	1.5	23	150	3	670
w/o added salt/low sodium	1/2 cup	6.0	1.5	11	110	3	25
Progresso sauces (canned)							
pasta, marinara, authentic	1/2 cup	4.0	1.0	12	100	3	590
pizza	1/2 cup	0.0	0.0	8	40	2	340
spaghetti	1/2 cup	4.5	1.0	12	100	2	620
Ragú sauces							
beef w/mushroom, Robusto!	1/2 cup	3.0	0.5	9	70	2	680
chunky garden, garden combination	1/2 cup	3.0	0.0	17	100	2	550
chunky garden, Mama's Special Garden	1/2 cup	3.0	0.5	18	110	2	530
chunky garden, mushroom & green pepper	1/2 cup	3.0	0.0	16	100	2	580
chunky garden, roasted red pepper & onion	1/2 cup	3.0	0.0	18	110	2	480
chunky garden, sundried tomato & basil	1/2 cup	3.0	0.0	18	110	2	510
chunky garden, super chunky mushroom	1/2 cup	3.0	0.0	18	110	2	520
chunky garden, super vegetable primavera	1/2 cup	3.0	0.0	16	100	2	490
chunky garden, tomato basil & cheese	1/2 cup	3.0	0.0	18	110	2	650
chunky garden, tomato	1/2 cup	3.0	0.0	18	110	2	520

	Serving	Total Fat (g)	Saturated Fat (g)	Total Carbohydrate (g)	Total Calories	Dietary Fiber	Sodium (mg)
garlic & onion							
old-world style, marinara	1/2 cup	4.5	0.5	11	80	2	780
old-world style, mushroom	1/2 cup	3.0	0.0	8	70	2	750
Parmesan & Romano, Robusto!	1/2 cup	3.5	0.5	10	90	2	570
pizza, homemade style	1/2 cup	2.0	0.0	8	60	2	520
roasted garlic primavera, light	1/2 cup	0.0	0.0	9	45	2	370
roasted garlic, Robusto!	1/2 cup	3.0	0.0	11	80	2	560
sautéed onion & mushroom, Robusto!	1/2 cup	4.0	0.5	9	80	2	610
7-herb tomato, Robusto!	1/2 cup	3.5	0.5	9	80		570
tomato & basil, light	1/2 cup	0.0	0.0	10	50	2	370
tomato & basil, no added sugar, light	1/2 cup	1.5	0.0	7	50	2	350
traditional, for snack, Pizza Quick	1/2 cup	4.0	0.0	8	80	2	760
Tomato Sauces and Pastes							
Contadina							
tomato paste	2 T.	0.0	0.0	6	30	1	20
tomato puree	1/4 cup	0.0	0.0	4	20	1	15
tomato sauce	1/4 cup	0.0	0.0	3	15	1	280
Del Monte							
tomato paste	2 T.	0.0	0.0	7	30	2	25
tomato sauce	1/4 cup	0.0	0.0	4	20	1	340
Hunt's							
tomato paste, pouch	2 T.	0.0	0.0	5	20	2	90
tomato puree	1/4 cup	0.0	0.0	6	25	2	25
Progresso							
tomato paste	2 T.	0.0	0.0	6	30	1	20
tomato puree	1/4 cup	0.0	0.0	5	25	1	15
tomato sauce, canned	1/4 cup	0.0	0.0	4	20	1	260
Gravies and Sauces							
Del Monte							
Sloppy Joe, original recipe	1/4 cup	0.0	0.0	16	70	0	680
Franco-American							
au jus	1/4 cup	0.5	0.0	2	10	0	310
beef	1/4 cup	1.5	0.5	3	30	0	310
beef, fat-free	1/4 cup	0.0	0.0	5	20	0	310

	Serving	Total Fat (g)	Saturated Fat (g)	Total Carbohydrate (g)	Total Calories	Dietary Fiber	Sodium (mg)
brown, w/onions	$^1/_4$ cup	1.0	0.0	4	25	0	340
chicken, fat-free	$^1/_4$ cup	0.0	0.0	3	15	0	320
mushroom	$^1/_4$ cup	1.0	0.0	3	20	0	300
turkey	$^1/_4$ cup	1.0	0.0	3	25	0	290
turkey, slow-roasted, fat-free	$^1/_4$ cup	0.0	0.0	6	30	0	370
Hunt's							
Sloppy Joe, Manwich	$^1/_4$ cup	0.0	0.0	6	30	1	380
Knorr							
au jus, prep w/water	$^1/_4$ cup	0.0	0.0	2	10	0	250
brown, classic, prep w/water	$^1/_4$ cup	0.5	0.0	3	20	0	380
brown, mushroom, prep w/water	$^1/_4$ cup	0.5	0.0	3	20	0	300
brown & onion, classic, prep w/water	$^1/_4$ cup	0.5	0.5	4	20	0	300
chicken, roasted, prep w/water	$^1/_4$ cup	0.5	0.0	4	25	0	340
hunter, prep w/water	$^1/_4$ cup	0.5	0.0	3	20	0	300
Lyonnaise, prep w/water	$^1/_4$ cup	0.5	0.5	4	20	0	300
pork, roasted, prep w/water	$^1/_4$ cup	0.0	0.0	4	25	0	230
turkey, roasted, prep w/water	$^1/_4$ cup	0.5	0.0	4	25	0	370
Pepperidge Farms							
Hearty Beef (jar)	$^1/_4$ cup	0.4	0.1	4	26	0	379

Baking Mixes

Criterion for general selection: ≤ 4 grams fat per serving

Brownie Mixes

	Serving	Total Fat (g)	Saturated Fat (g)	Total Carbohydrate (g)	Total Calories	Dietary Fiber	Sodium (mg)
Arrowhead Mills fat-free	$^1/_{16}$ pkg.	0.0	0.0	27	110	2	100
Krusteaz chocolate fudge, fat-free	$^1/_{16}$ pkg.	0.3	0.1	25	110	0	160
Snackwell's							
devil's food, low fat	$^1/_{16}$ pkg.	2.0	0.4	22	110	1	83
fudge, low fat	$^1/_{16}$ pkg.	2.0	0.4	23	120	1	90
Sweet Rewards, low fat	$^1/_{16}$ pkg.	2.5	1.0	27	130	1	115

Cake Mixes (prepared, w/o frosting)

	Serving	Total Fat (g)	Saturated Fat (g)	Total Carbohydrate (g)	Total Calories	Dietary Fiber	Sodium (mg)
Betty Crocker							
angel food	$^1/_{12}$ cake	0.0	0.0	27	120	0	200

	Serving	Total Fat (g)	Saturated Fat (g)	Total Carbohydrate (g)	Total Calories	Dietary Fiber	Sodium (mg)
gingerbread	1/12 cake	3.5	1.0	26	150	0	260
Krusteaz							
angel food	1/12 cake	0.0	0.0	32	140	0	370
devil's food	2×3" piece	3.5	1.0	27	150	1	280
lemon	2×3" piece	4.0	2.0	27	150	0	240
milk chocolate	2×3" piece	4.0	1.5	27	150	1	240
white or yellow	2×3" piece	3.5	1.0	27	150	0	240
Pillsbury							
angel food	1/12 cake	0.0	0.0	23	105	1	250
Snackwell's							
devil's food, low fat	1/12 cake	2.1	0.9	23	112	1	220
white or yellow, low fat	1/12 cake	2.1	0.6	23	120	1	185

Frostings, Syrups, and Toppings

Criterion for general selection: ≤ 2 grams fat per serving (~ 2 tablespoons)

Frostings

	Serving	Total Fat (g)	Saturated Fat (g)	Total Carbohydrate (g)	Total Calories	Dietary Fiber	Sodium (mg)
Snackwell/Pillsbury							
chocolate fudge, low fat	2 T.	3.0	1.0	22	120	0	65
milk chocolate	2 T.	3.0	1.0	22	120	1	80
white, fluffy, prep f/dry w/water	6 T.	0.0	0.0	25	100	0	60

Syrups

	Serving	Total Fat (g)	Saturated Fat (g)	Total Carbohydrate (g)	Total Calories	Dietary Fiber	Sodium (mg)
Hershey Foods							
chocolate	2 T.	0.4	0.3	24	102	1	19
chocolate, lite, tbsp	2 T.	0.2	0.0	12	51	0	35
chocolate malt	2 T.	0.3	0.0	25	106	1	68
Smucker's							
caramel	2 T.	0.0	0.0	25	100	0	105
caramel sundae	2 T.	0.0	0.0	25	100	0	110
chocolate, sugar free, fat free	2 T.	0.0	0.0	24	100	1	40
chocolate sundae	2 T.	0.0	0.0	26	110	0	20
strawberry sundae	2 T.	0.0	0.0	26	110	0	5
Three Musketeers sundae	2 T.	2.0	1.0	23	110	0	70

Toppings

	Serving	Total Fat (g)	Saturated Fat (g)	Total Carbohydrate (g)	Total Calories	Dietary Fiber	Sodium (mg)
Kraft							
butterscotch	2 T.	1.5	1.0	28	130	0	150
chocolate	2 T.	0.0	0.0	26	110	1	30
marshmallow crème	2 T.	0.0	0.0	10	40	0	10
pineapple	2 T.	0.0	0.0	28	110	0	15

	Serving	Total Fat (g)	Saturated Fat (g)	Total Carbohydrate (g)	Total Calories	Dietary Fiber	Sodium (mg)
strawberry	2 T.	0.0	0.0	29	110	0	15
Smucker's							
butterscotch caramel	2 T.	1.0	0.5	30	130	1	70
butterscotch, spoonable	2 T.	0.0	0.0	31	130	1	110
caramel, fat-free, microwave	2 T.	0.0	0.0	28	110	0	122
caramel, spoonable	2 T.	0.0	0.0	31	130	1	110
chocolate fudge, microwave	2 T.	1.5	0.5	28	130	1	60
chocolate fudge, spoonable	2 T.	1.5	0.5	28	130	1	60
dulce de leche	2 T.	1.5	1.0	23	110	0	45
hot fudge, fat-free, microwave	2 T.	0.0	0.0	26	100	1	70
hot fudge, light, spoonable	2 T.	0.0	0.0	23	90	2	95
hot fudge, sugar-free, fat-free	2 T.	0.0	0.0	24	100	1	40
pineapple, spoonable	2 T.	0.0	0.0	28	110	0	0
strawberry, spoonable	2 T.	0.0	0.0	26	100	0	0
Topping, whipped							
Cabot Creamery							
whipped cream	2 T.	2.0	1.5	2	30	0	0
Kraft							
extra creamy, Cool Whip	2 T.	2.0	2.0	2	25	0	5
fat-free, Cool Whip	2 T.	0.0	0.0	3	15	0	5
light, Cool Whip	2 T.	1.0	1.0	2	20	0	5
nondairy, Cool Whip	2 T.	1.5	1.5	2	25	0	0
prep w/milk & vanilla f/dry mix Dream Whip whipped	2 T.	1.0	0.5	2	20	0	5
	2 T.	1.5	1.0	1	20	0	0
PET whipped topping	2 T.	2.0	2.0	2	30	0	0
Reddi-Whip, fat-free	2 T.	0.5	0.2	2	13	0	6
Rich nondairy, ready to whip, prep f/fzn	2 T.	2.1	1.9	2	26	0	5

Pie Fillings, Puddings, Gelatins

Criterion for general selection: ≤ 3 grams fat per 1/2 cup serving

Pie Fillings (canned)

Comstock

	Serving	Total Fat (g)	Saturated Fat (g)	Total Carbohydrate (g)	Total Calories	Dietary Fiber	Sodium (mg)
apple	1/2 cup	0.0	0.0	30	120	0	15
blueberry	1/2 cup	0.0	0.0	28	110	0	15
blueberry, lite	1/2 cup	0.0	0.0	17	75	0	15
cherry	1/2 cup	0.0	0.0	28	110	0	15

	Serving	Total Fat (g)	Saturated Fat (g)	Total Carbohydrate (g)	Total Calories	Dietary Fiber	Sodium (mg)
cherry, lite	½ cup	0.0	0.0	19	75	0	15
chocolate	½ cup	3.0	1.0	26	130	0	240
lemon	½ cup	1.0	0.0	34	140	0	110
mincemeat	½ cup	1.0	0.0	39	150	1	180
peach	½ cup	0.0	0.0	26	110	0	20
pumpkin	½ cup	0.0	0.0	24	100	0	180
Libby's							
apple	⅓ cup	0.1	0.0	22	85	1	37
blueberry	½ cup	0.2	0.0	38	154	2	10
cherry	½ cup	0.1	0.0	24	98	1	15
lemon	⅓ cup	5.9	1.4	61	306	0	71
pumpkin	½ cup	0.8	0.0	30	136	3	174
Pudding							
Kraft D-Zerta							
chocolate, prep w/skim milk	½ cup	1.9	1.1	13	81	0	239
vanilla, prep w/skim milk	½ cup	1.7	1.0	12	81	0	303
Kraft Handi-Snacks							
chocolate, fat-free, snack cup	1 each	0.0	0.0	21	90	0	170
vanilla, fat-free, snack cup	1 each	0.0	0.0	21	90	0	180
Healthy Choice snack cups							
chocolate double fudge	1 each	2.0	0.5	21	110	0	125
chocolate raspberry	1 each	2.0	0.5	22	110	0	125
French vanilla	1 each	2.0	0.5	20	110	0	125
tapioca, French creme	1 each	2.0	0.5	21	110	0	125
Hunt's fat-free snack cups							
chocolate	1 each	0.0	0.0	22	100	0	150
tapioca	1 each	0.0	0.0	19	80	0	150
vanilla	1 each	0.0	0.0	18	80	0	140
Jell-O Americana							
rice, prep w/skim milk	½ cup	0.0	0.0	29	140	0	160
tapioca, fat-free, prep w/skim milk	½ cup	0.0	0.0	28	130	0	180
Jell-O Cook & Serve							
banana cream, prep w/2% milk	½ cup	2.5	1.5	26	140	0	240
butterscotch, prep w/2% milk	½ cup	2.5	1.5	30	160	0	190

	Serving	Total Fat (g)	Saturated Fat (g)	Total Carbohydrate (g)	Total Calories	Dietary Fiber	Sodium (mg)
chocolate, fat-free, prep w/skim milk	1/2 cup	0.0	0.0	29	130	0	170
chocolate, reduced cal., prep w/2% milk	1/2 cup	2.5	1.5	13	90	1	170
flan, prep w/2% milk	1/2 cup	2.5	1.5	26	140	0	65
lemon, prep w/2% milk	1/2 cup	2.0	0.5	29	140	0	75
milk chocolate, prep w/2% milk	1/2 cup	3.0	1.5	28	150	1	170
vanilla, fat-free, prep w/skim milk	1/2 cup	0.0	0.0	28	130	0	200
Jell-O instant							
banana cream, prep w/2% milk	1/2 cup	2.5	1.5	29	150	0	410
banana, reduced cal., prep w/skim milk	1/2 cup	0.0	0.0	12	70	0	410
butterscotch, prep w/2% milk	1/2 cup	2.5	1.5	29	150	0	450
butterscotch, reduced cal., prep w/skim milk	1/2 cup	0.0	0.0	12	70	0	400
chocolate, fat-free, prep w/skim milk	1/2 cup	0.0	0.0	31	140	1	410
chocolate fudge, prep w/2% milk	1/2 cup	3.0	1.5	31	160	1	440
chocolate fudge, reduced cal., prep w/skim milk	1/2 cup	0.0	0.0	14	80	1	390
chocolate, prep w/2% milk	1/2 cup	2.5	1.5	31	160	1	470
chocolate, reduced cal., prep w/skim milk	1/2 cup	0.0	0.0	14	80	1	390
devil's food, fat-free prep w/skim milk	1/2 cup	0.0	0.0	31	140	1	420
French vanilla, prep w/2% milk	1/2 cup	2.5	1.5	29	150	0	410
lemon, prep w/2% milk	1/2 cup	2.5	1.5	29	150	0	370
pistachio, prep w/2% milk	1/2 cup	3.0	1.5	29	160	0	410
vanilla, fat-free, prep w/skim milk	1/2 cup	0.0	0.0	29	140	0	410
vanilla, prep w/2% milk	1/2 cup	2.5	1.5	29	150	0	410
vanilla, reduced cal., prep w/skim milk	1/2 cup	0.0	0.0	12	70	0	400

	Serving	Total Fat (g)	Saturated Fat (g)	Total Carbohydrate (g)	Total Calories	Dietary Fiber	Sodium (mg)
Jell-O snack cups, fat-free							
chocolate	1 each	0.5	0.3	23	102	1	192
chocolate vanilla swirl	1 each	0.0	0.0	23	100	1	190
devil's food	1 each	0.0	0.0	23	100	1	210
rocky road	1 each	0.0	0.0	23	100	1	190
tapioca	1 each	0.0	0.0	23	100	0	240
vanilla	1 each	0.2	0.2	23	104	0	241

Cereals/Ready to Eat

Criterion for general selection: ≤ 2 grams fat and ≥ 2 grams dietary fiber per serving

	Serving	Total Fat (g)	Saturated Fat (g)	Total Carbohydrate (g)	Total Calories	Dietary Fiber	Sodium (mg)
Arrowhead Mills cereals							
amaranth flakes	1 cup	2.0	0.0	25	130	3	0
barley flakes, rolled	1/3 cup	1.0	0.0	28	110	5	0
bran flakes	1 cup	1.0	0.0	22	100	4	80
corn flakes	1 cup	0.0	0.0	30	130	2	65
kamyt flakes	1 cup	1.0	0.0	25	120	3	65
multigrain flakes	1 cup	1.5	0.0	29	140	3	130
Nature O's	1 cup	2.0	0.5	24	130	3	5
oat-bran flakes	1 cup	2.0	1.0	22	110	4	60
oat flakes, rolled	1/3 cup	2.5	0.5	23	130	4	0
puffed kamut	1 cup	0.0	0.0	11	50	2	0
puffed wheat	1 cup	0.5	0.0	20	90	2	0
rye flakes, rolled	1/3 cup	0.5	0.0	24	110	4	0
spelt flakes	1 cup	1.0	0.0	22	100	3	60
wheat flakes, rolled	1/3 cup	0.5	0.0	24	110	5	0
Barbara's Bakery cereals							
Breakfast O's	1 1/4 cup	2.0	0.0	22	110	3	115
corn flakes	1 cup	0.0	0.0	26	110	2	130
Grain Shop	2/3 cup	1.0	0.0	24	90	8	110
Honey Crunch'n Oats	3/4 cup	1.0	0.0	24	120	2	135
Organic Crispy Wheats	3/4 cup	0.5	0.0	25	110	3	190
Organic Weetabix	2 biscuits	1.0	0.0	28	120	4	130
Puffins, caramel	3/4 cup	1.0	0.0	26	100	6	150
Puffins, honey rice	3/4 cup	1.5	0.0	25	120	2	125
Puffins, original	3/4 cup	1.0	0.0	23	90	5	190
Puffins, peanut butter	3/4 cup	2.0	0.5	23	110	2	130
Shredded Oats	1 1/4 cup	2.5	0.5	46	220	5	260
Shredded Oats, vanilla almond	1 cup	3.0	0.5	42	220	4	210

	Serving	Total Fat (g)	Saturated Fat (g)	Total Carbohydrate (g)	Total Calories	Dietary Fiber	Sodium (mg)
Shredded Spoonfuls	³/₄ cup	1.5	0.0	24	120	4	200
Shredded Wheat	2 biscuits	1.0	0.0	31	140	5	0
Soy Essence	³/₄ cup	0.5	0.0	25	110	5	115
Toasted O's, apple cinnamon	³/₄ cup	1.0	0.0	24	110	2	80
Toasted O's, honey nut	³/₄ cup	2.0	0.0	23	120	2	75
General Mills cereals							
Basic 4	1 cup	2.8	0.4	42	200	3	315
Cheerios	1 cup	1.8	0.4	22	110	3	273
Cheerios, multigrain	1 cup	1.2	0.3	24	110	3	200
Chex, multibran	1 cup	1.2	0.2	40	165	6	322
Chex, wheat	1 cup	0.6	0.1	24	108	3	267
Crispy Wheaties 'N Raisins	1 cup	0.9	0.2	45	180	5	250
Fiber One	¹/₂ cup	0.8	0.1	24	60	14	128
Nature Valley fruit granola, low fat	²/₃ cup	3.0	0.5	44	210	3	210
Total, raisin bran	1 cup	1.1	0.2	41	170	5	239
Total, wheat	1 cup	1.0	0.2	30	130	3	255
Wheaties	1 cup	1.0	0.2	24	110	3	218
Health Valley Granola O's							
almond or apple-cinnamon, fat-free	³/₄ cup	0.0	0.0	26	120	3	10
Healthy Choice cereals							
Almond Crunch w/raisins	1 cup	2.6	0.4	43	200	5	215
Brown Sugar Squares	1 cup	0.8	0.1	36	150	4	1
Kashi cereals							
Go Lean	1 cup	1.7	0.0	38	170	13	47
Go Lean, Crunch	1 cup	3.0	0.2	36	200	8	207
Good Friends	1 cup	1.6	0.0	33	125	11	93
Heart to Heart	1 cup	2.1	0.0	33	150	6	116
Medley	¹/₂ cup	1.2	0.0	23	115	2	50
puffed	1 cup	0.5	0.0	20	90	2	0
Kellogg's cereals							
All-Bran, Bran Buds	¹/₃ cup	0.6	0.1	24	75	13	203
All-Bran, original	¹/₂ cup	1.0	0.2	24	80	10	80
All-Bran, w/extra fiber	¹/₂ cup	1.0	0.2	23	60	15	143
Apple Cinnamon or Blueberry Squares	³/₄ cup	1.0	0.2	44	180	5	20
Apple Raisin Crisp	1 cup	0.5	0.1	47	185	4	375

	Serving	Total Fat (g)	Saturated Fat (g)	Total Carbohydrate (g)	Total Calories	Dietary Fiber	Sodium (mg)
Common Sense oat bran flakes	1 cup	1.3	0.2	32	140	5	280
Complete wheat bran flakes	1 cup	0.8	0.1	30	120	7	270
Frosted Bran	1 cup	0.4	0.0	34	135	5	275
Frosted Mini Wheats	1 cup	0.8	0.2	41	175	5	5
Nutri-Grain, almond & raisin	1 cup	2.2	0.1	30	145	3	140
Nutri-Grain, wheat	1 cup	1.3	0.1	32	140	5	290
Raisin Bran Crunch	1 cup	1.0	0.2	45	188	4	210
Raisin Squares, mini wheats	³/₄ cup	0.9	0.2	44	185	5	3
Smart Start w/soy protein	1 cup	0.5	0.1	36	180	2	280
Strawberry Squares, mini wheats	1 cup	1.1	0.2	44	180	5	17
Nabisco cereals							
100% Bran	¹/₂ cup	1.6	0.3	24	90	10	228
Shredded Wheat, bite size, frosted	1 cup	1.0	0.2	44	180	5	10
Post cereals							
Blueberry Morning	1 cup	2.0	0.2	35	170	2	200
bran flakes	1 cup	1.0	0.2	32	130	7	290
Fruit & Fibre, peach raisin almond	1 cup	3.0	0.5	42	210	5	260
Grape-Nuts Flakes	1 cup	1.0	0.2	32	140	4	180
Grape-Nuts	¹/₂ cup	1.1	0.2	46	210	5	350
raisin bran	1 cup	1.1	0.2	46	190	8	360
Shredded Wheat, biscuits	2 each	0.6	0.1	38	160	5	3
Shredded Wheat 'N Bran	1 cup	0.6	0.1	38	160	6	3
Shredded Wheat, spoon size	1 cup	0.5	0.1	41	165	6	3
Quaker cereals							
Crunchy Bran	1 cup	1.3	0.3	32	120	6	310
Life, cinnamon	1 cup	2.0	0.4	40	190	3	240
Oatmeal Squares	1 cup	2.4	0.5	44	210	4	270
Shredded Wheat, biscuits	3 each	1.2	0.4	50	215	7	3
Shredded Wheat, small biscuits	1 cup	0.7	0.1	35	150	4	4
Toasted Oat Bran	1 cup	2.0	0.3	32	160	4	260
toasted oats	1 cup	1.5	0.3	23	115	2	285

	Serving	Total Fat (g)	Saturated Fat (g)	Total Carbohydrate (g)	Total Calories	Dietary Fiber	Sodium (mg)
Ralston							
40% Bran Flakes	1 cup	1.5	0.3	23	115	2	285
Muesli, blueberry pecan	1 cup	2.5	1.5	41	200	4	170
raisin bran	1 cup	0.3	0.0	47	180	8	485

Cereals/Cooked

Criterion for general selection: ≤ 2 grams fat and ≥ 1 gram fiber per serving (~1 cup prepared)

Cooked/Instant Cereals, prepared w/water & no added fat

	Serving	Total Fat (g)	Saturated Fat (g)	Total Carbohydrate (g)	Total Calories	Dietary Fiber	Sodium (mg)
Arrowhead Mills							
Bear Mush	1/4 cup dry	1.0	0.0	33	160	2	0
bulgur wheat	1/4 cup dry	0.5	0.0	33	150	4	0
cracked wheat	1/4 cup dry	0.5	0.0	29	140	6	0
four grain, plus flax	1/4 cup dry	2.0	0.0	28	150	6	0
oat bran	1/4 cup dry	1.9	0.0	17	115	5	0
oatmeal, instant, apple raisin almond	1 pkg.	2.0	0.0	24	130	2	0
oatmeal, instant, maple apple spice	1 pkg.	2.0	0.0	25	130	2	40
oatmeal, instant, original	1 pkg.	2.0	0.0	19	110	2	0
Rice & Shine	1/4 cup dry	1.0	0.0	32	150	2	0
seven grain	1/3 cup dry	1.5	0.0	25	140	5	0
Fantastic Foods hot cereal in a cup							
oatmeal, apple cinnamon	1 each	2.0	0.0	37	170	4	240
oatmeal, cranberry orange	1 each	2.0	0.0	38	180	4	210
peach berry wheat & oat	1 each	1.5	0.0	42	190	5	260
three grain, strawberry banana	1 each	2.0	0.0	53	240	5	292
wheat 'n berries	1 each	2.0	0.0	40	170	5	230
Hodgson Mill							
bulgur wheat with soy	1/4 cup dry	1.0	0.0	22	115	3	0
cracked wheat	1/4 cup dry	1.0	0.0	25	110	5	0
multigrain w/flax seed & soy	1/3 cup dry	3.0	0.5	25	160	6	0
oat bran	1/4 cup dry	3.0	1.0	23	120	6	3
wheat germ, untoasted	1/4 cup dry	2.0	0.0	14	110	8	0
Malt-O-Meal, plain	1/4 cup dry	0.4	0.1	32	150	2	3
Maypo	1/2 cup dry	2.0	0.4	34	180	5	9
Mother's/Quaker							
oat bran	1/2 cup dry	3.0	0.5	25	150	6	0

	Serving	Total Fat (g)	Saturated Fat (g)	Total Carbohydrate (g)	Total Calories	Dietary Fiber	Sodium (mg)
oatmeal, instant	1/2 cup dry	3.0	0.5	27	150	4	0
rolled oats	1/2 cup dry	3.0	0.5	27	150	4	0
whole wheat	1/2 cup dry	1.0	0.0	30	130	4	0
Nabisco							
Cream of Wheat	1/4 cup dry	0.6	0.1	33	160	2	3
Cream of Wheat, instant	1/4 cup dry	0.6	0.1	34	160	1	7
Cream of Wheat, mix 'n eat, flavored varieties	1 pkg.	0.4	0.1	29	130	1	240
Cream of Wheat, plain	1 pkg.	0.3	0.1	21	100	1	240
farina, Creamy Wheat	1/4 cup dry	0.4	0.1	34	150	1	1
Quaker							
grits, corn, instant, plain	1 pkg.	0.3	0.0	22	95	1	305
grits, hominy, quick	1/4 cup dry	0.5	0.1	29	125	2	1
grits, hominy, white, regular	1/4 cup dry	0.6	0.1	32	140	2	1
multigrain	1/2 cup dry	1.0	0.2	29	130	5	1
oatmeal, apple cinnamon, instant	1 pkg.	1.4	0.3	26	125	3	120
oatmeal, cinnamagic, instant	1 pkg.	2.0	0.4	31	155	3	255
oatmeal, cinnamon spice, instant	1 pkg.	2.1	0.4	36	170	3	242
oatmeal, maple & brown sugar, instant	1 pkg.	1.9	0.4	33	160	3	240
oatmeal, Quick 'N' Hearty, microwave							
brown sugar cinnamon	1 pkg.	2.2	0.4	31	155	3	255
cinnamon double raisin	1 pkg.	2.2	0.4	35	170	3	275
honey bran	1 pkg.	2.1	0.4	31	150	3	252
Ralston 100% wheat	1/4 cup dry	0.6	0.1	22	100	4	3
regular	1 pkg.	2.1	0.4	19	105	2	152
scotch barley	1/3 cup dry	1.1	0.2	37	165	5	3
whole wheat	1/2 cup dry	0.8	0.1	30	140	3	1
oatmeal, raisin cookie, instant	1 pkg.	2.1	0.4	32	155	2	225
oatmeal, raisins dates & walnuts, instant	1 pkg.	2.2	0.3	27	135	2	237
Roman Meal, plain	1/2 cup dry	1.0	0.2	33	150	8	3
Roman Meal, w/oats	1/2 cup dry	2.0	0.2	34	170	7	10

	Serving	Total Fat (g)	Saturated Fat (g)	Total Carbohydrate (g)	Total Calories	Dietary Fiber	Sodium (mg)
The Spice Hunter, apple cinnamon	1 cup	1.6	0.3	47	215	5	255
Wheatena	1/3 cup dry	1.3	0.2	35	165	6	6
Zoom, whole wheat	1/3 cup dry	0.6	0.1	23	125	7	2

Crackers, Croutons, Bread Sticks

Criterion for general selection: ≤ 2 grams fat per ounce (≤ 1 gram fat per 1/2 ounce)

Bread Sticks

	Serving	Total Fat (g)	Saturated Fat (g)	Total Carbohydrate (g)	Total Calories	Dietary Fiber	Sodium (mg)
Lance, all varieties	2 each	0.0	0.0	6	30	0	45
Stella D'Oro							
garlic or original	1 each	1.0	0.0	7	45	0	50
Grissini Style fat-free	3 each	0.0	0.0	12	60	0	130
Crackers							
B. Manischewitz matzoh							
Everything!/Onion & Poppy	1 each	0.5	0.0	22	110	1	150
Savory Garlic	1 each	0.0	0.0	23	100	1	200
unsalted/Tea Thins	1 each	0.0	0.0	24	110	1	0
whole wheat	1 each	0.5	0.0	22	110	4	0
Barbara's Bakery crackers							
Cheese Bites	26 each	2.0	0.3	24	120	1	290
Rite Lite Rounds	5 each	1.0	0.0	12	55	0	150
Breton, Reduced Fat & Sodium crackers	3 each	2.0	0.5	9	60	1	75
Carr's Table Water crackers, all varieties	5 each	1.5	0.0	13	70	0	60
Devonsheer Melba Rounds							
garlic, organic	5 each	1.0	0.0	11	60	1	85
honey bran, twelve grain	5 each	0.0	0.0	12	50	1	85
onion/vegetable	5 each	0.0	0.0	12	50	1	85
sesame, organic	5 each	2.0	0.5	10	60	1	125
Devonsheer Melba Toast							
sesame	3 each	1.0	0.0	11	50	1	90
other varieties	3 each	0.0	0.0	11	50	1	90
Finn Crisp crispbread							
light, Hi-Fiber	1 each	1.0	0.0	8	35	0	60
regular/dark/caraway	2 each	1.0	0.0	9	38	2	130
rye, Hi-Fiber	1 each	0.0	0.0	10	40	0	95

	Serving	Total Fat (g)	Saturated Fat (g)	Total Carbohydrate (g)	Total Calories	Dietary Fiber	Sodium (mg)
Frookie							
cracked pepper, low sodium fat-free	8 each	0.0	0.0	16	70	1	85
garlic & herb, fat-free	8 each	0.0	0.0	16	70	1	170
water, low sodium, fat-free	8 each	0.0	0.0	16	70	1	135
Hain crackers							
Bites, Golden Cheddar /White Cheddar	22 pieces	1.5	0.0	23	120	1	450
herb	11 each	0.0	0.0	23	110	1	190
saltine	5 each	0.0	0.0	0	60	0	130
soup/oyster	36 pieces	0.0	0.0	13	60	0	130
whole wheat	11 each	0.0	0.0	24	110	1	190
Health Valley fat-free crackers							
chili & cheese	6 each	0.0	0.0	11	50	2	80
graham, amaranth/oat bran	8 each	0.0	0.0	23	100	3	30
jalapeno cheese	6 each	0.0	0.0	11	50	2	80
pizza	6 each	0.0	0.0	11	50	2	140
whole wheat	5 each	0.0	0.0	11	50	2	80
whole wheat, low sodium	5 each	0.0	0.0	11	50	2	15
Healthy Choice Bread Crisp, garlic herb	11 each	2.0	0.5	22	110	2	115
Keebler crackers							
graham, crispy, low fat	4 each	1.7	0.4	23	115	1	115
graham, French vanilla, low fat	4 each	1.3	0.3	18	90	1	85
Zesta saltines, fat-free	5 each	0.0	0.0	13	60	0	250
Nabisco crackers							
Honey Maid, graham, cinnamon	8 each	2.0	0.5	24	120	0	170
Honey Maid, graham, honey/plain	8 each	2.0	0.5	22	120	0	180
Pepperidge Farm crackers							
Snackmix, Fat-Free Goldfish	2/3 cup	0.0	0.0	23	90	0	380
water, cracked pepper, biscuit type	5 each	1.0	0.5	12	60	1	90
water, original, biscuit type	5 each	1.0	0.5	11	60	1	100
Ry-Krisp crispbread, original	2 each	0.0	0.0	8	60	4	75

	Serving	Total Fat (g)	Saturated Fat (g)	Total Carbohydrate (g)	Total Calories	Dietary Fiber	Sodium (mg)
Snackwell's							
cheese	38 each	2.0	0.6	23	125	1	340
Classic Golden	6 each	1.0	0.2	11	60	0	145
salsa cheddar	32 each	2.0	0.5	23	120	1	340
wheat, fat-free	7 each	0.5	0.1	12	60	1	170
Sunshine, Krispy, fat-free	5 each	0.0	0.0	13	60	0	250
Wasa							
Crisp	3 each	0.0	0.0	11	50	2	100
Crispbread Cinnamon Toast	1 each	1.0	0.0	11	60	1	65
Crispbread Fiber Rye	1 each	1.0	0.0	4	30	2	60
Crispbread MultiGrain	1 each	0.0	0.0	8	45	2	85
Crispbread Whole Wheat	1 each	1.0	0.0	11	50	1	55
Crisp 'N Light Sourdough Rye	3 each	0.0	0.0	12	60	1	120
Crisp 'N Light Wheat	2 each	0.0	0.0	10	50	1	100
Westbrae rice wafers							
brown, no salt	7 each	0.5	0.0	11	50	0	0
brown, onion garlic	7 each	0.0	0.0	11	50	0	55
brown, sesame/tamari	7 each	0.0	0.0	11	50	0	70
Croutons							
Brownberry, toasted	2 T.	1.0	0.0	5	30	0	45
Devonsheer	2 T.	0.5	0.0	5	30	0	75
Old London	2 T.	1.0	0.0	5	30	1	85

Cookies

Criterion for general selection: ≤ 2 grams fat per ounce

	Serving	Total Fat (g)	Saturated Fat (g)	Total Carbohydrate (g)	Total Calories	Dietary Fiber	Sodium (mg)
Archway cookies							
cinnamon honey hearts, fat-free	3 each	0.2	0.1	25	105	0	123
devil's food, homestyle, fat-free	1 each	0.2	0.1	16	68	1	79
fruit bar, fat-free	1 each	0.0	0.0	21	90	0	95
lemon nuggets, fat-free	1 each	0.2	0.1	27	114	0	116
oatmeal raisin, homestyle, fat-free	1 each	0.5	0.0	24	106	1	164
pfeffernusse	1 each	0.5	0.0	16	70	0	50
raspberry oatmeal, homestyle, fat-free	1 each	0.5	0.1	25	108	1	166
sugar, homestyle, fat-free	1 each	0.2	0.1	17	70	0	80

	Serving	Total Fat (g)	Saturated Fat (g)	Total Carbohydrate (g)	Total Calories	Dietary Fiber	Sodium (mg)
Barbara's cookies							
apple-cinnamon filled, whole wheat	1 each	0.0	0.0	14	60	2	20
blueberry filled, traditional	1 each	1.0	0.0	14	60	1	25
fig filled, traditional	1 each	1.0	0.0	14	60	1	25
fig filled, whole wheat	1 each	0.0	0.0	16	60	2	20
Entenmann's cookies							
chocolate brownie, fat-free	2 each	0.0	0.0	20	80	1	90
chocolate, fudge brownie, fat-free	1 each	0.0	0.0	27	110	1	140
oatmeal chocolate chip, fat-free	2 each	0.0	0.0	19	80	1	110
oatmeal raisin, fat-free	2 each	0.0	0.0	18	80	1	120
oatmeal raisin, soft, light	2 each	0.0	0.0	23	100	2	135
Famous Amos cookies							
gingersnap, iced, low-fat	6 each	1.2	0.4	20	100	1	96
lemon snap, iced, low-fat	6 each	1.4	0.4	20	100	0	100
Frookie							
gingersnap, old fashioned	8 each	2.0	0.0	24	120	1	110
lemon wafer, fat-free	8 each	0.0	0.0	26	110	1	130
vanilla wafer, fat-free	8 each	0.0	0.0	26	110	0	120
Hain Cookie Jar Bites							
peanut butter	17 each	1.0	0.3	12	60	0	105
s'mores	17 each	0.0	0.0	12	60	0	20
Health Valley cookies							
apple bakes, fat-free	1 each	0.0	0.0	18	70	2	30
apple, fruit center, fat-free	1 each	0.0	0.0	18	70	2	20
apple raisin, fruit center, fat-free	1 each	0.0	0.0	18	70	2	20
apple raisin, jumbo, fat-free	1 each	0.0	0.0	19	80	3	35
apple spice, fat-free	3 each	0.0	0.0	24	100	3	50
apricot delight, fat-free	3 each	0.0	0.0	24	100	3	50
apricot, fruit center, fat-free	1 each	0.0	0.0	18	70	2	20
blueberry apple bakes, fat-free	1 each	0.0	0.0	26	110	3	25
chocolate chip, all varieties, fat-free	3 each	0.0	0.0	24	100	4	20
chocolate, fudge center, fat-free	2 each	0.0	0.0	17	70	3	20

Serving	Total Fat (g)	Saturated Fat (g)	Total Carbohydrate (g)	Total Calories	Dietary Fiber	Sodium (mg)
chocolate w/caramel center, 2 each fat-free	0.0	0.0	17	70	3	20
cobbler bites, all varieties 2 each	1.5	0.5	21	100	1	40
date bakes, fat-free 1 each	0.0	0.0	18	70	2	30
date bar, fat-free 1 each	0.0	0.0	34	140	3	50
date delight, fat-free 3 each	0.0	0.0	24	100	3	50
date, w/fruit center, fat-free 1 each	0.0	0.0	18	70	2	20
fruit, Hawaiian, fat-free 3 each	0.0	0.0	24	100	3	50
oatmeal raisin, fat-free 3 each	0.0	0.0	24	100	3	50
raisin bakes, fat-free 1 each	0.0	0.0	18	70	2	30
raisin bar, fat-free 1 each	0.0	0.0	35	140	3	5
raisin, jumbo, fat-free 1 each	0.0	0.0	19	80	3	35
raspberry, fruit center, 1 each fat-free	0.0	0.0	18	70	2	20
raspberry, jumbo, fat-free 1 each	0.0	0.0	19	80	3	35
raspberry/strawberry bakes, 1 each fat-free	0.0	0.0	26	110	3	25
strawberry granola bar, 1 each fat-free	0.0	0.0	35	140	3	5
tropical, w/fruit center, 1 each fat-free	0.0	0.0	18	70	2	20
LaChoy fortune cookies 4 each	0.2	0.0	26	112	1	11
Lance apple bar, fat-free 1 each	0.0	0.0	38	160	1	80
Nabisco cookies						
apple cinnamon Newton 1 each Cobblers	0.0	0.0	17	70	0	40
apple newton, fat-free 1 each	0.0	0.0	16	72	0	40
cranberry newton, fat-free 1 each	0.0	0.0	16	68	0	76
fig newton 1 each	1.5	0.5	10	60	1	60
fig newton, fat-free 1 each	0.0	0.0	16	70	0	76
gingersnap, old-fashioned 4 each	2.5	0.5	22	120	1	170
Nilla wafers, reduced fat 8 each	2.0	0.4	24	120	0	105
peach-apricot Newton 1 each Cobblers	0.0	0.0	17	70	0	55
raspberry or strawberry 1 each newton, fat-free	0.0	0.0	16	70	0	76
strawberry-kiwi Tropical 2 each	1.5	0.5	19	90	0	55

	Serving	Total Fat (g)	Saturated Fat (g)	Total Carbohydrate (g)	Total Calories	Dietary Fiber	Sodium (mg)
Newtons							
Nabisco Snackwells							
devil's food, fat-free	2 each	0.4	0.1	24	100	1	56
double fudge, fat-free	2 each	0.4	0.2	24	105	1	141
Stella D'oro cookies							
anisette sponge	2 each	1.0	0.0	19	90	0	80
anisette toast	3 each	1.0	0.0	27	130	0	150
egg biscuit, jumbo	2 each	1.0	0.0	18	90	0	60
fruit slices, fat-free	1 each	0.0	0.0	12	50	0	45
Sunshine Golden Fruit Biscuits	1 each	2.0	0.5	15	80	0	55
Sweet 'n Low cookies							
meringue, chocolate, sugar-& fat-free	14 each	0.0	0.0	26	80	1	0
meringue, vanilla, sugar-& fat-free	18 each	0.0	0.0	27	90	1	0

Packaged Snacks/Chips, Fruit Snacks, Pretzels, Popcorn, Rice Cakes
Criterion for general selection: ≤ 3 grams fat per 1- ounce serving

Chips, Puffs, and Snacks

	Serving	Total Fat (g)	Saturated Fat (g)	Total Carbohydrate (g)	Total Calories	Dietary Fiber	Sodium (mg)
Arrowhead Mills Corn Curls							
blue corn	1 oz.	2.0	0.0	22	120	4	54
blue corn, unsalted	1 oz.	2.0	0.0	22	120	4	1
yellow corn	3/4 oz.	1.0	0.0	18	90	3	31
yellow corn w/cheese	3/4 oz.	2.0	0.5	15	90	3	30
Barbara's Bakery Pinta Puffs, salsa corn chips	1 oz.	2.0	0.0	10	70	0	130
Bugles Light & Baked Corn Snacks	1 cup	3.0	0.0	16	90	0	280
Doritos WOW tortilla chips	1 oz.	1.0	0.0	18	90	1	240
Genisoy Soy Crisps, varieties avg.	1 oz.	2.0	0.0	15	100	2	250
Guiltless Gourmet							
baked potato chips	1 oz.	1.5	0.0	22	110	1	200
tortilla chips	1 oz.	2.0	0.0	22	110	2	140
Hain							
baked potato crisps	1 oz.	1.5	0.0	23	110	0	150
cheese puffs, fat-free	1 oz.	0.0	0.0	22	105	2	245
corn puffs, fat-free	1 oz.	0.0	0.0	23	105	2	55
Health Valley nonfat caramel puffs	1 cup	0.0	0.0	24	110	2	60

	Serving	Total Fat (g)	Saturated Fat (g)	Total Carbohydrate (g)	Total Calories	Dietary Fiber	Sodium (mg)
Lay's							
baked potato chips, varieties avg.	1 oz.	1.5	<1.0	23	110	0	150
WOW potato chips	1 oz.	0.0	0.0	18	75	0	200
Louise's potato chips							
nonfat varieties	1 oz.	0.0	0.0	23	110	2	180
original	1 oz.	1.0	0.0	23	100	0	200
Ruffles							
baked potato chips	1 oz.	3.0	1.0	21	120	0	200
WOW potato chips	1 oz.	0.0	0.0	17	75	0	200
Skinny Natural Corn Chips							
barbeque	1 cup	1.0	0.0	12	60	1	140
nacho flavor	1 cup	1.0	0.0	12	60	1	105
no salt	1 cup	1.0	0.0	12	60	1	0
salted	1 cup	1.0	0.0	12	60	1	58
sour cream & onion	1 cup	1.0	0.0	12	65	1	70
Tostitos							
baked	1 oz.	1.0	0.0	24	110	2	200
WOW	1 oz.	1.0	0.0	20	90	1	105
Fruit Snacks							
Criterion for general selection: ≤3 grams fat per ounce							
Betty Crocker							
Fruit by the Foot, grape or strawberry	1 each	1.5	0.5	17	80	0	45
Fruit Roll-Up, berry with vit. C	1 each	0.5	0.0	12	50	0	44
Fruit Roll-Up, grape	1 each	0.7	0.2	12	55	0	58
Fun Snacks, berry n' blue, cherry, strawberry, stripes	1 pouch	1.0	0.0	21	90	0	23
Gushers, all flavors	1 pouch	1.0	0.0	20	90	0	55
Brach's							
Hi-C fruit snacks	1 pouch	0.0	0.0	19	80	0	35
Minute Maid, all-natural fruit snacks	1 pouch	0.0	0.0	17	70	0	10
Specialty shapes	1 pouch	1.0	0.0	18	80	0	25
Farley Candy Co. Fruit snacks, w/vit. A, C, & E	1 each	0.0	0.0	21	90	0	9
Kellogg							
Fruit Twistables	1 each	0.5	0.0	18	80	0	75

	Serving	Total Fat (g)	Saturated Fat (g)	Total Carbohydrate (g)	Total Calories	Dietary Fiber	Sodium (mg)
Nabisco							
CapriSun, fruit punch	1 pouch	2.0	1.0	16	80	0	0
Jell-O fruit snacks	1 pouch	0.0	0.0	19	80	0	15
Sunbelt Fruit Jammers	1 ounce	1.0	0.0	24	105	0	30
Sunkist Fruit Roll	1 each	0.0	0.0	18	70	1	20
Popcorn, Microwave varieties (as consumed)							
Cracker Jacks							
butter toffee or caramel, fat-free	3 cups	0.0	0.0	26	110	1	71
Healthy Choice, butter or natural flavor	3 cups	3.0	0.0	26	120	5	330
Jolly Time							
butter flavor, light	3 cups	2.0	1.0	12	60	3	105
natural flavor, light	3 cups	2.0	1.0	13	70	3	110
Newman's Own Oldstyle Picture Show, light	3½ cups	3.0	1.0	20	110	3	90
Orville Redenbacher's							
butter-flavored light, snack size	3 cups	3.0	1.0	11	70	1	90
hot air, Gourmet	3 cups	1.0	0.0	10	40	3	0
Smart Pop butter flavored	3 cups	1.0	0.0	11	50	1	100
Smart Pop kettle korn	3 cups	1.5	0.0	14	60	3	180
Pop-Secret							
butter flavor, light	3 cups	3.0	1.0	12	70	2	95
light	3 cups	2.5	1.0	10	60	2	150
94% fat-free	3 cups	1.0	0.0	12	55	2	115
Pop Weaver							
butter light	3 cups	2.5	0.5	12	75	2	150
Kettle Korn	3 cups	3.0	1.0	13	90	2	150
Weight Watchers	1-oz. pkg.	1.0	0.0	22	100	1	5
Pretzels							
Bachman							
traditional varieties averaged	1 oz.	1.0	0.0	23	110	1	820
fat-free varieties	1 oz.	0.0	0.0	23	110	1	125
Frito Lay Rold Gold							
sticks, thins, & tiny twists, fat-free	1 oz.	0.0	0.0	23	110	1	530
Pepperidge Farms							
Goldfish, pretzel flavor	1 oz.	2.0	0.5	21	115	1	405

	Serving	Total Fat (g)	Saturated Fat (g)	Total Carbohydrate (g)	Total Calories	Dietary Fiber	Sodium (mg)
traditional	1 oz.	3.0	0.0	21	120	1	400
variety pack, on the go	1 each	2.5	0.5	20	110	1	400
Snyder's							
mini, olde tyme, thins	1 oz.	0.0	0.0	23	110	0	330
rods, snaps	1 oz.	1.0	0.0	24	120	0	400
Rice/Popcorn Cakes							
Lundberg Family							
rice cake, brown	1 each	0.5	0.0	16	75	0.5	57
rice cake, multigrain	1 each	0.0	0.0	15	65	1	22
rice cake, popcorn, organic	1 each	0.0	0.0	12	60	0.5	35
rice cake, salted	1 each	0.5	0.0	15	70	0.5	54
Quaker							
rice cake, chocolate crunch	1 each	1.0	0.5	12	60	0.5	35
rice cake, cinnamon streusel	1 each	1.0	0.0	12	60	0	22
rice cake, peanut butter	1 each	1.0	0.0	12	60	0	61
rice cake, plain	1 each	0.0	0.0	8	35	0	14
rice cake, plain, unsalted	1 each	0.0	0.0	7	35	0	0
Westbrae, varieties averaged	1 each	0.0	0.0	5	25	36	20

Packaged Snacks/Cakes and Pastries

Criterion for general selection: ≤ 4 grams fat per 2 ounces

	Serving	Total Fat (g)	Saturated Fat (g)	Total Carbohydrate (g)	Total Calories	Dietary Fiber	Sodium (mg)
Entenmann's							
buns, fat-free (varieties averaged)	1 each	0.0	0.0	33	150	1	140
cake, iced, fat-free (varieties averaged)	1 piece	0.0	0.0	50	210	2	247
cake, Louisiana Crunch, fat-free	1 piece	0.0	0.0	51	220	1	220
cake, no icing, fat-free (varieties averaged)	1 piece	0.0	0.0	33	140	2	164
loaf, fat-free (varieties averaged)	1 piece	0.0	0.0	31	130	1	230
pastry, fat-free (varieties averaged)	1 piece	0.0	0.0	40	170	1	140
pie, fat-free (varieties averaged)	1 piece	0.0	0.0	65	270	2	320
Health Valley							
brownie—2 varieties (avg.)	1 each	0.0	0.0	26	110	4	30
snack bar, breakfast—7 varieties (avg.)	1 each	0.0	0.0	26	110	3	25

	Serving	Total Fat (g)	Saturated Fat (g)	Total Carbohydrate (g)	Total Calories	Dietary Fiber	Sodium (mg)
snack bar, cereal—3 varieties (avg.)	1 each	0.0	0.0	26	150	3	38
snack bar, chocolate—4 varieties (avg.)	1 each	0.0	0.0	26	150	3	35
snack bar, marshmallow—3 varieties (avg.)	1 each	0.0	0.0	22	90	1	0
snack bar, rice—3 varieties (avg.)	1 each	0.0	0.0	26	110	1	5
tart—7 varieties (avg.)	1 each	0.0	0.0	35	150	3	30
Little Debbie							
reduced-fat brownie	1 each	3.0	1.0	39	190	1	200
reduced fat oatmeal crème pie	1 each	2.5	2.5	29	130	0	180
Nutri-Grain bars, multiple flavors (avg.)	1 each	2.5	0.5	27	136	<1	110
Quaker Oats breakfast bars							
fruit flavors & oatmeal (avg.)	1 each	3.0	0.4	26	135	1	118
low-fat granola	1 each	2.0	0.8	22	110	1	80
Snackwell's							
fruit-filled cereal bar	1 each	0.0	0.0	29	120	1	105

Nutrition/Sports Bars and Shakes

Criterion for general selection: ≤ 6 grams fat per serving (2 ounce bar or 8 ounce shake)

Nutrition/Sports Bars

	Serving	Total Fat (g)	Saturated Fat (g)	Total Carbohydrate (g)	Total Calories	Dietary Fiber	Sodium (mg)
Balance bars (varieties averaged)	1 bar	6.0	3.0	23	200	1	180
Clif bars (varieties averaged)	1 bar	5.0	1.5	45	250	5	150
Dr. Soy protein bars (varieties averaged)	1 bar	4.5	2.5	25	180	1	130
Genisoy soy protein bars (varieties averaged)	1 bar	5.0	3.0	35	240	2	170
Kashi GoLEAN bars (varieties averaged)	1 bar	5.5	4.0	49	290	6	200
Luna bars (varieties averaged)	1 bar	4.0	2.5	25	180	2	125
PowerBar bars							
Harvest (varieties averaged)	1 bar	4.0	0.5	45	240	4	80
Harvest, dipped (varieties averaged)	1 bar	5.0	2.0	45	250	2	125

	Serving	Total Fat (g)	Saturated Fat (g)	Total Carbohydrate (g)	Total Calories	Dietary Fiber	Sodium (mg)
Performance (varieties averaged)	1 bar	2.5	0.5	45	235	3	110
Pria (varieties averaged)	1 bar	3.0	2.0	16	110	1	80
Promax bars (varieties averaged)	1 bar	6.0	3.0	40	285	1	180
Slim-Fast bars							
Breakfast & Lunch Bars (varieties averaged)	1 bar	5.5	3.0	20	145	2	75
Chewy Granola Bars (varieties averaged)	1 bar	5.5	3.0	35	220	1	220
High Protein Bars (varieties averaged)	1 bar	6.0	4.0	25	210	1	240
Layered Bars (varieties averaged)	1 bar	5.0	4.0	34	220	2	180
Meal On-the-Go Bars (varieties averaged)	1 bar	5.0	3.0	35	220	2	125
Nutrition & Meal Replacement Shakes							
Boost, canned, chocolate vanilla	8 oz.	4.0	1.0	40	240	0	130or
Carnation (varieties averaged)							
Instant Breakfast, prep w/skim milk	9 oz.	1.5	0.8	39	220	1	240
Instant Breakfast, w/o added sugar, prep w/skim milk	9 oz.	1.5	0.8	24	160	1	220
ready-to-drink, canned	10 oz.	2.5	1.0	35	210	1	210
Ensure, canned (varieties averaged)	8 oz.	6.0	1.0	35	250	0	200
Genisoy soy protein shakes, powder	1 scoop	0.0	0.0	18	125	2	175
Slim-Fast							
Ready-to-Drink (varieties averaged)	11 oz.	3.0	1.0	40	220	5	220
Ready-to-Drink w/Soy (varieties averaged)	11 oz.	1.0	0.0	46	220	5	180
Sustacal, canned (varieties averaged)	8 oz.	6.0	1.0	33	240	<1	220

	Serving	Total Fat (g)	Saturated Fat (g)	Total Carbohydrate (g)	Total Calories	Dietary Fiber	Sodium (mg)

Candy

Criterion for general selection: ≤ 1 gram fat per 1-ounce serving (28 grams)

NOTE: Candy is made primarily from refined sugars and contains minimal nutrients

Brach's candies

	Serving	Total Fat (g)	Saturated Fat (g)	Total Carbohydrate (g)	Total Calories	Dietary Fiber	Sodium (mg)
candy corn	26 pieces	0.0	0.0	35	140	0	80
cinnamon Imperials	52 pieces	0.0	0.0	15	60	0	0
gumdrops	12 pieces	0.0	0.0	32	130	0	0
hard, all flavors	1 piece	0.0	0.0	6	25	0	3
hard, sugar-free, all flavors	1 piece	0.0	0.0	3	10	0	0
jelly beans	14 pieces	0.0	0.0	38	150	0	5
lemon drops	4 pieces	0.0	0.0	18	70	0	5
licorice	5 pieces	1.5	0.0	38	150	0	65
orange slices, Hi-C	2 pieces	0.0	0.0	15	60	0	6
red laces	3 strands	1.0	0.0	40	160	0	10
Star Brites peppermint	3 pieces	0.0	0.0	15	60	0	0
Breath Savers, all flavors	1 piece	0.0	0.0	3	10	0	0
Campfire marshmallows	6 large	0.0	0.0	28	110	0	15
Hershey Twizzlers, cherry bits	18 pieces	0.5	0.0	30	120	0	85
Hershey Twizzlers, strawberry twists	3 pieces	0.5	0.0	30	120	0	85
Jolly Ranchers, all flavors	3 pieces	0.0	0.0	18	70	0	10
Kraft candies							
buttermints	7 pieces	0.0	0.0	15	60	0	25
jet-puffed marshmallows	5 pieces	0.0	0.0	28	110	0	40
marshmallow crème	2 T.	0.0	0.0	10	40	0	10
party mints	7 pieces	0.0	0.0	15	60	0	35
Lifesavers, all flavors	2 pieces	0.0	0.0	5	20	0	0
Lifesavers, Gummi Savers	11 pieces	0.0	0.0	32	130	0	0
Mars candies							
Skittles	10 pieces	0.5	0.1	10	45	0	2
Starburst fruit chews	2 pieces	0.8	0.1	8	40	0	6
Nestle SweeTarts	8 pieces	0.0	0.0	14	60	0	0
Now & Laters, all flavors	6 pieces	1.0	0.5	25	110	0	40
Tootsie Roll pop	1 pop	0.0	0.0	15	60	0	10

Dairy Foods/Milk, Cream, Sour Cream

Criterion for general selection: ≤ 2 grams fat per 1 cup (8 ounces) serving

Sour Cream and Cream: ≤ 1 gram fat per tablespoon

Condensed Milk

Eagle

	Serving	Total Fat (g)	Saturated Fat (g)	Total Carbohydrate (g)	Total Calories	Dietary Fiber	Sodium (mg)
sweetened fat-free	2 T.	0.1	0.0	24	109	0	41
sweetened low fat	2 T.	1.5	1.0	23	117	0	39
Cream/Cream Substitutes							
Carnation Coffee-Mate nondairy							
fat-free, flavored	1 T.	0.0	0.0	5	25	0	0
fat-free, plain	1 T.	0.0	0.0	5	25	0	0
light	1 T.	0.5	0.0	2	15	0	0
regular	1 T.	0.0	0.0	2	7	0	0
Eagle nondairy creamer	1 t.	0.3	0.1	2	9	0	3
International Delight nondairy creamers	1 T.	0.0	0.0	7	30	0	5
Rich's Poly Rich							
coffee rich	1 T.	0.5	0.2	2	12	0	8
farm rich	1 T.	0.8	0.3	1	10	0	6
Silk soy milk creamer							
French vanilla	1 T.	1.0	0.0	3	20	0	5
hazelnut	1 T.	1.0	0.0	1	16	0	5
plain	1 T.	1.0	0.0	1	15	0	5
Dry Milk							
Carnation nonfat dry milk	1/3 cup	0.0	0.0	12	80	0	125
Saco cultured buttermilk	1/4 cup	<1.0	0.0	13	80	0	166
Evaporated Milk							
Carnation							
low-fat	2 T.	0.5	0.5	3	25	0	35
nonfat	2 T.	0.0	0.0	4	25	0	40
Pet evaporated nonfat milk	2 T.	0.0	0.0	4	25	0	40
Milk							
Darigold skim milk	1 cup	0.0	0.0	14	100	0	140
USDA averages							
buttermilk, low fat	1 cup	2.2	1.3	12	98	0	260
chocolate, low fat	1 cup	1.2	0.7	27	144	2	120
nonfat/skim	1 cup	0.5	0.3	12	90	0	130
1/2% low fat	1 cup	1.0	0.5	12	90	0	125
Soy Milk							
Edensoy, light, plain	1 cup	2.0	0.0	14	90	0	85
Galaxy chocolate veggie soy milk	1 cup	2.0	0.0	26	150	2	130
Health Valley fat-free soy milk	1 cup	0.0	0.0	22	110	1	60

	Serving	Total Fat (g)	Saturated Fat (g)	Total Carbohydrate (g)	Total Calories	Dietary Fiber	Sodium (mg)
Vitasoy							
cocoa light	1 cup	2.0	0.0	25	130	2	130
original light	1 cup	2.0	0.0	15	90	2	95
vanilla light	1 cup	2.0	0.0	20	110	2	95
Westsoy							
lite, chocolate	1 cup	1.5	0.0	25	120	2	55
lite, plain	1 cup	1.5	0.0	15	90	2	90
lite, vanilla	1 cup	1.5	0.0	19	110	2	65
low fat, plain	1 cup	1.5	0.0	14	90	2	90
low fat, vanilla	1 cup	1.5	0.0	21	120	2	90
nonfat, plain	1 cup	0.0	0.0	10	70	<1	105
nonfat, vanilla	1 cup	0.0	0.0	12	80	<1	105
Sour Cream							
Breakstone's fat-free	2 T.	0.5	0.3	5	174	0	208
Cabot non-fat	2 T.	0.0	0.0	3	20	0	40
Darigold nonfat	2 T.	0.0	0.0	4	25	0	50
Knudsen fat-free	2 T.	0.0	0.0	6	35	0	25
Land O' Lakes							
light sour cream	2 T.	2.0	1.5	4	35	0	30
nonfat sour cream	2 T.	0.0	0.0	5	30	0	40

Dairy Foods/Cheese

Criterion for general selection: ≤ 4 grams of fat per ounce

Cheeses

	Serving	Total Fat (g)	Saturated Fat (g)	Total Carbohydrate (g)	Total Calories	Dietary Fiber	Sodium (mg)
Alpine Lace							
feta, 50% less fat	1 oz.	3.0	2.0	1	50	0	370
feta w/tomato & basil, 50% less fat	1 oz.	3.0	2.0	1	50	0	370
goat cheese, 50% less fat	1 oz.	3.0	2.0	1	40	0	130
mozzarella low moisture, 50% less fat	1 oz.	3.0	2.0	1	70	0	200
Parmesan fat-free	2 T.	0.0	0.0	0	30	0	195
Healthy Choice							
American white singles	1 each	1.0	0.5	2	40	0	200
American yellow singles	1 each	1.0	0.5	2	40	0	200
cheddar, fancy, shredded	1/4 cup	1.5	1.0	1	50	1	220
cheddar, sharp singles	1 each	1.0	0.5	2	40	0	220
cheddar string cheese	1 each	1.5	1.0	1	50	0	220
garlic & herb, shredded	1/4 cup	1.5	1.0	1	50	1	260

	Serving	Total Fat (g)	Saturated Fat (g)	Total Carbohydrate (g)	Total Calories	Dietary Fiber (g)	Sodium (mg)
garlic & sundried tomato/ garlic lovers shredded	¼ cup	1.5	1.0	1	50	0	260
Italian fancy shredded	¼ cup	1.5	1.0	1	50	0	210
jalapeño singles	1 each	1.0	0.5	3	40	1	200
Mexican fancy shredded	¼ cup	1.5	1.0	1	50	0	220
mozzarella 1" cube	1 oz.	0.0	0.0	1	43	1	189
mozzarella fancy shredded	¼ cup	1.5	1.0	1	50	0	220
mozzarella fat-free shredded	¼ cup	0.0	0.0	2	45	0	200
pizza fancy shredded	¼ cup	1.5	1.0	1	50	1	220
Swiss low-fat singles	1 each	1.0	0.5	2	40	0	200
Kraft Cheeses							
cheddar fat-free shredded	¼ cup	0.0	0.0	1	40	0	270
Cheese Whiz light	2 T.	3.3	2.2	6	75	0	597
Free Singles, non-fat pasteurized processed	1 each	0.0	0.0	3	35	0	300
grated topping fat-free	2 T.	0.0	0.0	9	45	0	225
Healthy Favorites fat-free mozzarella shredded	¼ cup	0.0	0.0	2	45	1	340
mozzarella, shredded low fat	¼ cup	3.8	2.0	0.8	61	0	160
Singles, American cheese	1 each	3.0	2.0	2	50	0	320
Velveeta light	1 oz.	3.0	2.0	3	63	0	450
Lifeline fat-free cheeses							
1" cubes	1 oz.	0.0	0.0	1	40	0	220
shredded	¼ cup	0.0	0.0	2	34	0	235
Sargento mozzarella sticks low fat	1 each	2.5	1.5	1	50	0	180
Cheese Spreads							
Healthy Choice fat-free cream cheese							
herb & garlic	2 T.	0.0	0.0	2	25	1	200
strawberry	2 T.	0.0	0.0	5	35	1	200
Healthy Choice plain cream cheese fat-free	2 T.	0.0	0.0	2	25	1	200
Philadelphia							
soft fat-free	2 T.	0.0	0.0	2	30	0	200
soft garden vegetable fat-free	2 T.	0.0	0.0	2	30	0	220
soft w/strawberries fat-free	2 T.	0.0	0.0	6	45	0	190

	Serving	Total Fat (g)	Saturated Fat (g)	Total Carbohydrate (g)	Total Calories	Dietary Fiber	Sodium (mg)
Price's pimiento cheese spread light	2 T.	3.5	1.0	3	60	0	260
Cottage Cheese							
Breakstone							
dry curd 1/2% fat	1/2 cup	0.0	0.0	3	45	0	30
fat-free	1/2 cup	0.0	0.0	6	80	0	440
2% fat	1/2 cup	2.5	1.5	4	90	0	390
Darigold							
nonfat	1/2 cup	0.0	0.0	6	90	0	460
pineapple	1/2 cup	4.0	2.5	17	150	0	410
2% fat	1/2 cup	2.5	1.5	5	100	0	470
Knudsen							
nonfat	1/2 cup	0.0	0.0	4	80	0	380
1.5% fat w/peaches	4 oz.	1.5	1.0	13	110	0	300
1.5% fat w/pineapple	4 oz.	2.0	1.0	14	120	0	330
1.5% fat w/strawberries	4 oz.	1.5	1.0	13	110	0	290
1.5% fat w/tropical fruit	4 oz.	2.0	1.5	13	110	0	300
small curd 2% fat	1/2 cup	2.5	1.5	5	100	0	400
Light n' Lively							
nonfat	1/2 cup	0.0	0.0	6	80	0	440
1% fat garden salad w/calcium	1/2 cup	0.5	1.0	5	80	0	390
1% fat peach & pineapple w/ calcium	1/2 cup	1.0	0.5	15	110	0	340
1% fat w/ calcium	1/2 cup	1.0	1.0	5	80	0	370
Ricotta Cheese							
Sargento							
fat-free	1/4 cup	0.0	0.0	5	50	0	65
reduced fat	1/4 cup	2.5	1.5	3	60	0	55

Dairy Foods/Yogurt

Criterion for general selection: ≤ 2 grams of fat per cup (8 ounces)

	Serving	Total Fat (g)	Saturated Fat (g)	Total Carbohydrate (g)	Total Calories	Dietary Fiber	Sodium (mg)
Breyers							
low fat 1%, fruit flavors	8 oz.	2.0	1.5	45	240	0	125
nonfat, fruit flavors	8 oz.	0.0	0.0	22	120	0	105
Colombo							
classic	8 oz.	2.0	1.5	42	220	0	115
fruit on the bottom	8 oz.	2.0	1.5	47	230	0	90
light	8 oz.	0.0	0.0	21	120	0	110

	Serving	Total Fat (g)	Saturated Fat (g)	Total Carbohydrate (g)	Total Calories	Dietary Fiber (g)	Sodium (mg)
Danimals							
low fat, fruit flavors	4 oz.	0.5	0.0	21	110	0	85
Dannon							
light, flavors	8 oz.	0.5	0.0	33	170	0	180
nonfat, flavors	8 oz.	0.0	0.0	22	120	0	135
Double Delight low fat, flavored	8 oz.	1.0	0.5	38	180	0	170
Jell-O low fat 1% yogurts	8 oz.	1.0	0.5	25	130	0	65
Light n' Lively							
low fat 1%, fruit flavors	8 oz.	1.0	0.5	25	130	0	65
nonfat, fruit flavors	8 oz.	0.0	0.0	13	70	0	55
Silk soy yogurts	8 oz.	2.0	0.0	30	160	1	20
Yoplait							
lemon burst, Original	6 oz.	1.5	1.0	36	180	0	80
Light, fruit flavors	6 oz.	0.0	0.0	19	100	0	85
Light, indulgent flavors	6 oz.	0.0	0.0	19	100	0	90
Nouriche	11 oz.	0.0	0.0	60	290	6	290
Original, fruit flavors	6 oz.	1.5	1.0	33	170	0	80

Egg Substitutes

Criterion for general selection: ≤ 2 grams of fat per egg equivalent (¹/₄ cup)

	Serving	Total Fat (g)	Saturated Fat (g)	Total Carbohydrate (g)	Total Calories	Dietary Fiber (g)	Sodium (mg)
Fleischmann's Egg Beaters	¹/₄ cup	0.0	0.0	1	30	0	125
Healthy Choice	¹/₄ cup	<1.0	0.0	1	30	0	90
Morningstar Farms Better 'N Eggs							
frozen	¹/₄ cup	0.4	0.1	0	27	0	98
liquid	¹/₄ cup	0.0	0.0	1	25	0	81
Morningstar Farms Scramblers, frozen	¹/₄ cup	0.4	0.0	2	39	0	121
Tofutti Egg Watchers	¹/₄ cup	0.0	0.0	1	30	0	80

Fats/Reduced-Fat Margarines, Butter Substitutes, and Cooking Sprays

Criterion for general selection: ≤ 6 gram of fat per tablespoon

Butter Substitutes

	Serving	Total Fat (g)	Saturated Fat (g)	Total Carbohydrate (g)	Total Calories	Dietary Fiber (g)	Sodium (mg)
Butter Buds							
mix, liquefied	1 T.	0.0	0.0	2	5	0	75
sprinkles	1 t.	0.0	0.0	2	5	0	120
Molly McButter fat-free sprinkles							
butter flavor	1 t.	0.0	0.0	1	5	0	180
cheese flavor	1 t.	0.0	0.0	1	5	0	125

Cooking Sprays (1-second spray)

	Serving	Total Fat (g)	Saturated Fat (g)	Total Carbohydrate (g)	Total Calories	Dietary Fiber (g)	Sodium (mg)
Baker's Joy		0.5	0.0	0	5	0	0

	Serving	Total Fat (g)	Saturated Fat (g)	Total Carbohydrate (g)	Total Calories	Dietary Fiber	Sodium (mg)
Crisco (various flavors)		0.0	0.0	0	0	0	0
Hunt-Wesson		0.0	0.0	0	0	0	0
I Can't Believe It's Not Butter (various flavors)		0.0	0.0	0	0	0	0
Mazola		0.0	0.0	0	0	0	0
Pam (various flavors)		0.0	0.0	0	0	0	0
Parkay		0.0	0.0	0	0	0	5
Smart Balance		0.5	0.0	0	7	0	0
Reduced-Fat Margarines							
Benecol Light	1 T.	5.0	0.5	0	45	0	110
Blue Bonnet Light							
soft spread	1 T.	4.5	1.0	<1	40	0	90
stick	1 T.	5.0	1.0	<1	50	0	80
Brummel & Brown	1 T.	5.0	1.0	0	45	0	90
Fleischmann's Light							
soft spread	1 T.	4.5	0.0	0	40	0	90
stick	1 T.	5.0	1.0	<1	50	0	80
I Can't Believe It's Not Butter Light	1 T.	5.0	1.0	0	50	0	85
Parkay Light							
soft spread	1 T.	5.0	1.0	0	50	0	130
stick	1 T.	5.0	1.0	0	50	0	75
Promise							
Buttery Light	1 T.	5.0	1.0	0	45	0	55
fat-free margarine	1 T.	0.0	0.0	0	5	0	90
Shedd's Country Crock Light Spread	1 T.	5.0	1.0	0	50	0	85
Smart Balance Light Spread	1 T.	5.0	1.5	0	45	0	90
Smart Beat—Smart Squeeze (Nonfat spread)	1 T.	5.0	0.0	0	5	0	100
Take Control Light	1 T.	5.0	0.5	0	45	0	85

Fats/Reduced-Fat Mayonnaise and Salad Dressings
Criterion for general selection: ≤ 3 grams fat per 2-tablespoon serving

Mayonnaise Dressings							
Hellmann's low fat	1 T.	1.0	0.3	4	25	0	140
Kraft Free	1 T.	0.4	0.1	2	10	0	120
Miracle Whip fat-free	1 T.	0.4	0.1	3	15	0	125
Smart Beat fat-free	1 T.	0.0	0.0	3	10	0	135

Salad Dressings

	Serving	Total Fat (g)	Saturated Fat (g)	Total Carbohydrate (g)	Total Calories	Dietary Fiber	Sodium (mg)
Good Seasons							
honey French, fat-free, prep f/dry mix	2 T.	0.0	0.0	5	20	0	250
honey mustard, fat-free, prep f/dry mix	2 T.	0.0	0.0	5	20	0	280
Italian, fat-free, prep f/dry mix	2 T.	0.0	0.0	3	10	0	290
zesty herb, fat-free, prep f/dry mix	2 T.	0.0	0.0	2	10	0	260
Kraft Free							
blue cheese, fat-free	2 T.	0.0	0.0	11	45	1	360
Caesar, classic, fat-free	2 T.	0.0	0.0	11	45	1	360
Caesar Italian, fat-free	2 T.	0.0	0.0	4	25	0	480
Catalina, fat-free	2 T.	0.0	0.0	8	35	1	320
French, fat-free	2 T.	0.0	0.0	11	45	1	300
honey Dijon, fat-free	2 T.	0.0	0.0	10	45	1	330
Italian, creamy, fat-free	2 T.	0.0	0.0	12	50	1	330
Italian, fat-free	2 T.	0.3	0.2	4	20	0	430
ranch, fat-free	2 T.	0.4	0.1	11	48	0	354
ranch, garlic, fat-free	2 T.	0.0	0.0	11	45	1	320
ranch, peppercorn, fat-free	2 T.	0.0	0.0	11	45	1	330
ranch, sour cream & onion, fat-free	2 T.	0.0	0.0	11	50	1	300
red wine vinegar, fat-free	2 T.	0.0	0.0	3	15	0	410
thousand island, fat-free	2 T.	0.0	0.0	9	40	1	280
Kraft Light Done Right							
Catalina	2 T.	3.0	1.0	11	60	0	350
Italian	2 T.	3.0	1.0	3	40	0	270
Marie's							
blue cheese, creamy, low fat	2 T.	1.5	0.0	7	45	1	270
Italian, herb, creamy, low fat	2 T.	2.0	0.0	6	40	0	290
Parmesan, creamy, low fat	2 T.	1.5	0.0	7	45	0	270
ranch, zesty, low fat	2 T.	1.5	0.0	7	45	0	330
vinaigrette, classic herb, fat-free	2 T.	0.0	0.0	7	30	0	250

	Serving	Total Fat (g)	Saturated Fat (g)	Total Carbohydrate (g)	Total Calories	Dietary Fiber	Sodium (mg)
vinaigrette, honey Dijon, fat-free	2 T.	0.0	0.0	11	50	0	125
vinaigrette, Italian, fat-free	2 T.	0.0	0.0	8	35	0	280
vinaigrette, raspberry, fat-free	2 T.	0.0	0.0	8	35	0	35
vinaigrette, red wine, fat-free	2 T.	0.0	0.0	10	40	0	300
vinaigrette, white wine, fat-free	2 T.	0.0	0.0	10	40	0	310
Seven Seas							
Italian, creamy, fat-free	2 T.	0.0	0.0	12	50	1	330
Italian, Viva, fat-free	2 T.	0.0	0.0	2	10	0	480
ranch, fat-free	2 T.	0.0	0.0	11	45	1	330
raspberry vinaigrette, fat-free	2 T.	0.0	0.0	7	30	0	320
red wine vingear, fat-free	2 T.	0.0	0.0	3	15	0	410
Wishbone							
blue cheese, chunky, fat-free	2 T.	0.0	0.0	7	35	0	290
blue cheese, Just 2 Good	2 T.	2.0	1.0	6	45	0	320
Caesar, Just 2 Good	2 T.	2.0	1.0	5	40	0	310
French, Just 2 Good	2 T.	2.0	1.0	9	50	0	240
honey Dijon, Just 2 Good	2 T.	2.0	1.0	8	50	0	250
Italian, fat-free	2 T.	0.0	0.0	2	10	0	280
Italian, Just 2 Good	2 T.	2.0	1.0	5	35	0	480
ranch, Just 2 Good	2 T.	2.0	1.0	5	40	0	270
red wine vinaigrette, fat-free	2 T.	0.0	0.0	7	35	0	230
thousand island, Just 2 Good	2 T.	2.0	1.0	9	60	0	300

Condiments

Criterion for general selection: ≤ 1 gram of fat per tablespoon
Barbecue Sauce (NOTE: all brands meet criterion)
Catsup (NOTE: all brands meet criterion)
Cocktail Sauce (NOTE: all brands meet criterion)

Dips

	Serving	Total Fat (g)	Saturated Fat (g)	Total Carbohydrate (g)	Total Calories	Dietary Fiber	Sodium (mg)
Bearitos fat-free black bean dip	2 T.	0.0	0.0	4	25	1	150
Breakstone's fat-free dips creamy salsa	2 T.	0.0	0.0	3	20	0	240

	Serving	Total Fat (g)	Saturated Fat (g)	Total Carbohydrate (g)	Total Calories	Dietary Fiber	Sodium (mg)
French onion dip	2 T.	0.0	0.0	4	25	0	260
ranch dip	2 T.	0.0	0.0	4	25	0	330
Frito Lay dips							
bean dip	2 T.	1.0	0.5	6	40	0	140
hot bean dip	2 T.	1.0	0.0	5	40	1	170
Garden of Eatin' dips							
Baja black bean dip	2 T.	0.0	0.0	5	25	1	80
red bean spicy chipotle	2 T.	0.0	0.0	5	25	2	90
Guiltless Gourmet dips							
mild black bean dip	2 T.	0.0	0.0	5	30	1	100
spicy black bean dip	2 T.	0.0	0.0	5	30	1	100
spicy pinto bean dip	2 T.	0.0	0.0	6	35	2	100
Knudsen Free fat-free dips							
creamy salsa	2 T.	0.0	0.0	3	20	0	240
French onion dip	2 T.	0.0	0.0	4	25	0	260
ranch dip	2 T.	0.0	0.0	4	25	0	330
Kraft fat-free dips							
French onion dip	2 T.	0.0	0.0	4	25	0	260
ranch dip	2 T.	0.0	0.0	4	25	0	330
salsa	2 T.	0.0	0.0	3	20	0	240
Marzetti fat-free dips							
caramel apple dip	2 T.	0.0	0.0	28	120	0	115
chocolate fruit dip	2 T.	0.0	0.0	25	100	0	150
dill veggie dip	2 T.	0.0	0.0	6	30	0	410
ranch veggie dip	2 T.	0.0	0.0	6	35	0	320
sour cream & onion veggie dip	2 T.	0.0	0.0	6	35	0	300
southwestern ranch veggie dip	2 T.	0.0	0.0	6	30	0	380
Old El Paso Dips							
black bean dip	2 T.	0.0	0.0	5	25	1	280
jalapeño dip	2 T.	1.0	0.0	4	30	2	125
low-fat medium cheese 'n salsa	2 T.	1.5	1.0	3	30	0	240
Ortega frozen chunky fiesta salsa & beef	2 T.	2.0	1.0	5	50	1	170
Taco Bell fat-free black bean dip	2 T.	0.0	0.0	6	28	2	207

	Serving	Total Fat (g)	Saturated Fat (g)	Total Carbohydrate (g)	Total Calories	Dietary Fiber	Sodium (mg)

Mustards (NOTE: all brands meet criterion—exception is mayonnaise blends)
Steak Sauces (NOTE: all brands meet criterion)
Taco, Salsa, and Picante Sauces (NOTE: all brands meet criterion)
Tartar Sauce

	Serving	Total Fat (g)	Saturated Fat (g)	Total Carbohydrate (g)	Total Calories	Dietary Fiber	Sodium (mg)
Kraft fat-free tartar sauce	2 T.	0.0	0.0	5	25	0	200

Frozen Foods/Entrees and Meals

Criteria for general selection: ENTREES: ≤ 8 grams fat per 1-cup serving (minimum 5 ounces); MEALS: ≤ 12 grams fat per meal (minimum 10 ounces) and ≤ 1000 mg. sodium per serving

Beef/Pork Dinners and Entrees

	Serving	Total Fat (g)	Saturated Fat (g)	Total Carbohydrate (g)	Total Calories	Dietary Fiber	Sodium (mg)
Banquet sliced beef w/gravy, mashed potatoes, & peas	1 meal	10.0	4.3	19	270	4	742
Café Classics, Lean Cuisine							
beef peppercorn	1 meal	7.0	2.5	25	220	3	690
beef portobello	1 meal	7.0	3.0	25	220	3	690
beef pot roast	1 meal	6.0	2.0	25	200	2	690
honey-roasted pork	1 meal	4.0	1.5	34	230	3	690
meatloaf & whipped potatoes	1 meal	8.0	3.0	30	270	3	540
orange beef	1 meal	7.0	2.0	42	300	2	690
Oriental beef	1 meal	3.0	1.0	33	210	2	580
oven-roasted beef	1 meal	8.0	3.5	18	210	2	690
Salisbury steak	1 meal	9.0	4.5	24	270	3	680
Southern beef tips	1 meal	5.0	2.0	37	250	3	680
Dinnertime Selections, Lean Cuisine							
beef steak tips Dijon	1 meal	7.0	3.0	44	310	5	820
Salisbury steak	1 meal	9.0	4.5	35	320	6	890
Everyday Foods, Lean Cuisine							
steak tips portobello	1 entree	4.0	1.5	13	130	3	550
stuffed cabbage	1 entree	5.0	2.0	26	190	4	620
Swedish meatballs	1 entree	7.0	3.0	36	290	2	640
Freezer Queen sliced beef w/gravy & veg	1 meal	4.8	1.3	26	207	4	648
Healthy Choice							
beef merlot	1 meal	8.0	2.0	25	240	6	600
beef ribs w/classic barbecue sauce	1 meal	9.0	3.0	47	360	8	580
beef Stroganoff	1 meal	9.0	3.0	40	330	7	600
beef tips portobello	1 meal	8.0	3.0	28	280	3	600

	Serving	Total Fat (g)	Saturated Fat (g)	Total Carbohydrate (g)	Total Calories	Dietary Fiber (g)	Sodium (mg)
charbroiled beef patty	1 meal	9.0	3.0	40	310	6	600
grilled steak in roasted garlic sauce	1 meal	7.0	2.5	22	220	5	600
grilled whiskey steak	1 meal	6.0	2.0	38	280	6	600
oven-roasted beef	1 meal	7.0	2.5	33	280	5	600
pot roast	1 meal	9.0	3.0	39	320	6	550
Salisbury steak & red skin potatoes	1 meal	6.0	2.5	20	200	4	600
steak w/barbecue sauce	1 meal	9.0	3.0	57	410	11	600
steak w/teriyaki dipping sauce	1 meal	10.0	3.0	74	490	6	590
steak w/zesty steak sauce	1 meal	10.0	3.0	37	340	6	600
traditional meat loaf	1 meal	9.0	3.0	36	300	6	600
Healthy Choice Medleys							
beef teriyaki	1 meal	7.0	2.5	44	310	5	600
Stouffer's							
beef w/roasted potatoes & peppers	1 meal	6.0	1.5	44	300	7	830
homestyle pot roast	1 meal	9.0	3.0	30	200	4	790
Stouffer's Skillet Sensations							
beef & rice fiesta skillet	1 serving	3.5	1.5	48	300	6	760
beef teriyaki skillet	1 serving	5.0	1.5	52	320	4	890
savory beef & vegetables skillet	1 serving	7.0	3.0	38	290	9	760
Swanson							
beef & broccoli	1 meal	10.0	5.0	53	350	4	830
Yankee-style pot roast	1 meal	4.5	1.5	39	250	5	850
The Budget Gourmet							
beef pepper steak	1 meal	6.0	1.5	35	230	2	840
beef Stroganoff, low fat	1 meal	6.0	2.5	32	240	3	690
roast beef supreme	1 meal	10.0	4.0	34	270	2	690
Breakfasts							
Amy's Kitchen breakfast burrito	1 each	6.0	0.0	38	210	5	540
Lean Pockets							
bacon, egg, & cheese	1 each	4.5	1.0	21	150	2	280
sausage, egg, & cheese	1 each	4.5	1.5	19	140	2	310
Morningstar Farms vegetarian							
breakfast sandwich	1 each	3.0	0.5	35	280	5	1000

	Serving	Total Fat (g)	Saturated Fat (g)	Total Carbohydrate (g)	Total Calories	Dietary Fiber	Sodium (mg)
Swanson Great Start breakfast burritos							
ham & cheese	1 each	6.0	2.0	30	210	0	500
hot & spicy	1 each	7.0	3.0	30	220	3	490
original w/scrambled egg	1 each	8.0	3.0	25	200	2	510
Swanson Kid Breakfast Blast, pancakes	1 each	8.0	4.0	54	320	2	640
Chicken/Turkey Meals and Entrees							
Café Classics Bowls							
creamy chicken & vegetables	1 bowl	6.0	2.5	45	310	3	810
grilled chicken Caesar	1 bowl	5.0	1.5	30	240	4	710
Café Classics, Lean Cuisine							
baked chicken	1 meal	4.5	1.0	32	230	2	690
chicken à l'orange	1 meal	1.5	0.5	35	230	2	340
chicken & vegetables	1 meal	5.0	2.5	33	250	3	690
chicken carbonara	1 meal	7.0	2.0	31	270	2	690
chicken marsala	1 meal	4.0	1.5	12	140	3	620
chicken Mediterranean	1 meal	4.0	0.5	38	260	4	690
chicken Parmesan	1 meal	5.0	1.5	36	270	2	520
chicken piccata	1 meal	6.0	1.5	41	270	1	670
chicken w/almonds	1 meal	4.0	0.5	38	260	2	640
chicken w/basil cream sauce	1 meal	7.0	2.5	30	260	2	570
glazed chicken	1 meal	5.0	1.0	25	230	1	520
glazed turkey tenderloins	1 meal	6.0	1.5	39	270	4	610
grilled chicken	1 meal	5.0	1.0	15	160	4	690
herb-roasted chicken	1 meal	3.5	1.0	23	190	3	610
honey mustard chicken	1 meal	4.0	1.5	37	260	1	640
roasted garlic chicken	1 meal	5.0	1.5	28	230	1	640
roasted turkey breast	1 meal	2.5	0.5	51	270	3	690
sesame chicken	1 meal	8.0	1.5	48	320	2	690
sweet & sour chicken	1 meal	2.5	0.5	51	290	1	290
teriyaki chicken	1 meal	3.5	1.5	42	280	0	660
Thai-style chicken	1 meal	4.5	2.5	35	250	1	660
Dinnertime Selections, Lean Cuisine							
chicken fettuccine	1 meal	8.0	3.5	51	380	5	870
chicken Florentine	1 meal	6.0	2.5	53	370	6	870
glazed chicken	1 meal	6.0	1.0	39	310	3	650

	Serving	Total Fat (g)	Saturated Fat (g)	Total Carbohydrate (g)	Total Calories	Dietary Fiber	Sodium (mg)
grilled chicken & penne pasta	1 meal	6.0	2.5	46	340	5	680
grilled chicken Tuscan	1 meal	6.0	1.5	34	270	3	610
Oriental glazed chicken	1 meal	2.0	0.5	58	330	2	850
roasted chicken	1 meal	4.5	1.0	48	320	4	730
roasted turkey breast	1 meal	7.0	1.0	50	340	6	840
Everyday Foods, Lean Cuisine							
baked chicken Florentine	1 meal	4.0	1.0	25	190	2	690
honey Dijon grilled chicken	1 meal	8.0	2.0	25	230	3	690
roasted chicken	1 meal	7.0	2.0	33	260	2	670
roasted turkey & vegetables	1 meal	2.0	0.5	13	120	4	450
three-cheese chicken	1 meal	7.0	2.5	15	190	2	580
Healthy Choice							
chicken Margherita	1 meal	8.0	1.5	42	340	6	600
chicken teriyaki	1 meal	6.0	2.0	37	270	6	600
chicken Tuscany	1 meal	9.0	3.0	39	340	4	600
chicken w/honey barbecue sauce	1 meal	9.0	2.0	46	390	5	580
chicken w/honey mustard	1 meal	5.0	1.0	49	360	6	600
chicken w/roasted red pepper sauce	1 meal	10.0	3.5	47	420	4	570
chicken w/teriyaki sauce	1 meal	9.0	2.0	66	470	4	600
chicken w/tomato garlic sauce	1 meal	9.0	2.0	47	410	5	600
country breaded chicken	1 meal	9.0	3.0	55	370	5	600
country herb chicken	1 meal	6.0	2.5	37	280	5	600
grilled basil chicken	1 meal	9.0	3.0	37	330	5	600
grilled chicken Caesar	1 meal	8.0	2.5	33	300	5	600
grilled chicken marinara	1 meal	4.5	1.5	35	270	5	580
grilled turkey breast	1 meal	5.0	2.0	31	250	5	600
honey glazed chicken	1 meal	6.0	2.0	46	320	6	580
mesquite barbecue chicken	1 meal	5.0	2.0	44	300	5	480
princess chicken	1 meal	7.0	2.0	41	310	5	580
roasted chicken breast	1 meal	8.0	3.0	32	280	7	600
roasted chicken Chardonnay	1 meal	8.0	3.0	32	290	4	600
traditional turkey breast	1 meal	5.0	2.0	50	330	4	600
Healthy Choice Duos							
breaded chicken strips w/mac & cheese	1 meal	5.0	2.0	35	290	3	600

	Serving	Total Fat (g)	Saturated Fat (g)	Total Carbohydrate (g)	Total Calories	Dietary Fiber	Sodium (mg)
grilled chicken breast & mashed potatoes	1 meal	5.0	1.5	19	190	3	580
grilled chicken breast & pasta	1 meal	7.0	2.5	25	250	4	560
slow-roasted turkey breast	1 meal	7.0	1.5	17	210	4	600
Healthy Choice Medley							
chicken breast & vegetables	1 meal	7.0	2.0	30	260	6	550
chicken carbonara	1 meal	7.0	2.5	39	310	2	600
chicken piccata	1 meal	5.0	2.5	36	260	2	600
country glazed chicken	1 meal	5.0	2.0	28	230	3	600
Mandarin chicken	1 meal	3.5	0.5	36	250	4	520
roast turkey breast	1 meal	6.0	2.0	23	220	2	580
Stouffer's baked chicken w/rice & vegetable	1 meal	8.0	2.0	55	410	4	850
Stouffer's Skillet Sensations							
chicken Alfredo	1 serving	4.0	2.0	23	180	2	480
chicken Oriental	1 serving	3.0	0.5	23	170	2	610
chicken primavera	1 serving	2.5	0.5	28	180	4	430
chicken teriyaki	1 serving	3.0	1.0	37	230	2	620
garlic chicken	1 serving	4.5	2.0	36	240	2	580
herb chicken & roasted potatoes	1 serving	3.0	0.5	24	170	2	510
roasted turkey	1 serving	1.5	0.5	23	130	3	450
three-cheese chicken	1 serving	5.0	2.0	26	200	2	460
Swanson							
chicken & noodle casserole	1 entree	9.0	3.0	36	300	2	940
grilled chicken w/garlic	1 meal	6.0	3.0	35	260	5	660
herb roasted chicken	1 meal	7.0	2.5	44	310	3	780
The Budget Gourmet							
French recipe chicken	1 meal	5.6	1.4	10	180	6	865
glazed turkey tenderloins	1 entrée	5.0	2.0	43	260	5	660
Mandarin chicken	1 entree	6.0	1.5	38	240	2	780
orange glazed chicken	1 entree	3.5	1.0	54	300	2	440
Oriental chicken & vegetables	1 entree	6.0	1.5	42	260	3	590
teriyaki chicken w/oriental vegetables	1 dinner	3.7	0.6	52	320	4	675
Tyson							
mesquite barbecue chicken	1 meal	7.8	2.6	45	320	4	795

	Serving	Total Fat (g)	Saturated Fat (g)	Total Carbohydrate (g)	Total Calories	Dietary Fiber (g)	Sodium (mg)
roasted chicken w/garlic sauce	1 meal	6.7	1.3	22	215	4	470
Weight Watchers barbecue glazed chicken	1 meal	4.4	1.0	26	220	0	405
Weight Watchers Smart Ones roast turkey medallions & mushrooms	1 meal	2.0	0.0	35	215	3	504
Chinese Dinners and Entrees							
Amy's Kitchen							
Asian noodle stir fry	1 entrée	4.5	0.5	41	240	4	680
teriyaki bowl	1 bowl	2.0	0.0	59	300	3	780
Bird's Eye							
Chinese vegetable stir fry	1 meal	0.5	0.1	19	90	5	605
teriyaki vegetable stir fry	1 meal	1.1	0.3	17	90	1	720
Café Classics bowls							
chicken teriyaki	1 bowl	2.5	0.5	63	340	2	790
fried rice	1 bowl	8.0	1.5	64	410	4	890
teriyaki steak	1 bowl	7.0	2.5	48	340	4	890
Chun King sweet & sour chicken	1 entrée	1.8	0.5	32	165	1	565
Everyday Foods, Lean Cuisine							
chicken chow mein	1 entrée	3.5	1.0	35	230	2	670
Hunan beef & broccoli	1 entrée	4.0	1.5	36	230	1	680
Mandarin chicken	1 entrée	3.5	1.0	46	270	2	690
Oriental style pot stickers	1 entrée	6.0	2.0	55	320	3	610
teriyaki stir fry	1 meal	4.5	1.0	49	300	3	690
vegetable eggroll	1 each	6.0	1.5	62	330	3	720
Green Giant Create-a-Meal							
Oriental style pasta w/vegetables	2½ cups	10.0	4.0	35	260	4	580
vegetable lo mein stir fry	2⅓ cup	1.0	0.0	35	170	4	920
vegetable sweet & sour stir fry	1¾ cup	0.0	0.0	29	130	5	390
vegetable teriyaki stir fry	1¾ cup	0.5	0.0	18	100	4	850
Healthy Choice							
Oriental style beef	1 meal	9.0	2.5	33	310	5	580
Oriental style chicken	1 meal	5.0	1.5	28	240	4	600
sesame chicken	1 meal	6.0	2.0	34	260	4	580
sweet & sour chicken	1 meal	7.0	2.0	54	340	3	580

	Serving	Total Fat (g)	Saturated Fat (g)	Total Carbohydrate (g)	Total Calories	Dietary Fiber	Sodium (mg)
La Choy							
chicken teriyaki	³/₄ cup	2.3	0.5	11	82	2	915
chow mein, beef	1 cup	1.7	0.8	15	105	4	755
chow mein, chicken	1 cup	3.6	0.9	11	90	2	865
egg roll, chicken, mini	3 each	4.5	1.2	12	105	1	325
Oriental beef pepper steak	1 cup	2.4	0.6	13	104	4	970
The Budget Gourmet							
Chinese vegetables w/chicken, rice & sauce	1 entree	6.0	2.5	40	250	3	670
spicy Szechuan style vegetables w/chicken & pasta	1 entree	9.0	2.0	41	280	3	880
Fish/Shellfish Dinners and Entrees							
Café Classics, Lean Cuisine							
baked fish w/pasta shells & vegetables	1 meal	6.0	3.0	40	290	2	690
shrimp & angel hair pasta	1 meal	5.0	1.0	34	240	2	680
Healthy Choice							
herb baked fish	1 meal	8.0	2.0	55	360	5	590
lemon pepper fish	1 meal	5.0	2.0	49	280	5	580
shrimp & vegetables	1 meal	6.0	3.0	39	270	6	580
tuna casserole	1 meal	7.0	1.5	31	270	5	600
Italian/Pasta Meals and Entrees							
Amy's Kitchen							
cannelloni w/vegetables	1 meal	12.0	8.0	34	330	6	600
garden vegetable lasagna	1 entree	9.0	4.0	41	290	5	720
pasta w/vegetables & Parmesan sauce	1 cup	8.0	4.0	27	220	4	460
tofu vegetable lasagna	1 entrée	10.0	1.5	41	300	6	630
Banquet lasagna w/meat sauce	8-oz. serving	10.0	6.0	33	270	2	960
Café Classics, Lean Cuisine							
bow tie pasta & chicken	1 meal	4.0	1.0	31	220	3	680
cheese lasagna w/chicken	1 meal	8.0	2.0	36	280	3	490
Café Classics bowl							
three-cheese stuffed rigatoni	1 bowl	6.0	3.0	46	280	4	680
Dinnertime Selections, Lean Cuisine							
jumbo rigatoni	1 meal	10.0	3.5	50	390	6	790

	Serving	Total Fat (g)	Saturated Fat (g)	Total Carbohydrate (g)	Total Calories	Dietary Fiber	Sodium (mg)
Everyday Foods, Lean Cuisine							
Alfredo pasta w/chicken & broccoli	1 meal	6.0	3.0	38	270	3	690
angel hair pasta	1 meal	4.0	1.5	48	260	4	690
cheese cannelloni	1 meal	4.5	2.0	31	240	3	240
cheese lasagna Florentine bake	1 meal	7.0	4.5	37	270	3	680
cheese ravioli	1 meal	6.0	3.0	38	250	3	620
chicken fettuccine	1 meal	6.0	3.0	34	270	2	690
chicken Florentine lasagna	1 meal	6.0	2.5	36	270	3	690
classic five-cheese lasagna	1 meal	7.0	4.0	44	310	4	660
fettuccine Alfredo	1 meal	7.0	3.5	40	280	2	670
lasagna w/meat sauce	1 meal	7.0	3.0	43	310	3	650
macaroni & beef	1 meal	6.0	2.0	38	270	3	660
macaroni & cheese	1 meal	7.0	4.0	42	300	1	650
penne pasta w/tomato	1 meal	3.5	1.0	50	270	5	390
spaghetti w/meat sauce	1 meal	5.0	1.5	35	240	3	690
spaghetti w/meatballs	1 meal	5.0	2.0	37	260	3	590
Healthy Choice frozen meals							
chicken broccoli Alfredo	1 meal	7.0	3.0	34	300	2	530
chicken Parmigiana	1 meal	9.0	3.0	40	320	6	600
Healthy Choice Medleys							
chicken fettuccine Alfredo	1 meal	7.0	2.5	32	290	3	570
rigatoni w/broccoli & chicken	1 meal	7.0	2.5	29	270	5	600
Healthy Choice Solos							
fettuccine Alfredo	1 meal	7.0	2.5	40	280	3	580
lasagna bake	1 meal	7.0	2.5	38	270	4	600
macaroni & cheese	1 meal	7.0	3.0	44	290	5	600
manicotti w/three cheeses	1 meal	5.0	3.0	44	280	4	600
spaghetti w/meat sauce	1 meal	6.0	2.5	48	310	7	600
stuffed pasta shells	1 meal	4.0	2.0	41	270	9	470
Morton's spaghetti w/meat sauce	1 meal	6.0	2.5	30	200	4	750
The Budget Gourmet frozen meals							
angel hair pasta w/tomatoes in meat sauce	1 meal	5.0	1.5	39	240	3	450
fettuccine & meatballs w/sauce & green beans	1 meal	7.0	3.0	42	280	2	560

	Serving	Total Fat (g)	Saturated Fat (g)	Total Carbohydrate (g)	Total Calories	Dietary Fiber	Sodium (mg)
fettuccine primavera w/chicken & herb sauce	1 meal	7.0	2.0	30	230	2	540
Italian vegetables w/chicken, rice, & sauce	1 entree	6.0	2.0	39	250	2	540
lasagna, mozzarella	1 entree	8.0	3.0	45	300	3	590
lasagna w/meat sauce	1 entree	9.0	3.0	40	300	3	490
lasagna w/meat sauce, low fat	1 entree	7.0	3.0	34	250	3	580
linguini w/clams & bay shrimp, marinara	1 entree	8.0	2.5	44	290	2	450
linguini w/clams & shrimp, low fat	1 entree	6.0	2.5	41	270	2	440
pasta primavera, low fat	1 entree	6.0	2.5	36	240	4	540
pasta w/chicken in wine & mushroom sauce	1 entree	7.0	2.0	41	280	4	670
penne pasta w/tomato, sausage, & sauce	1 entree	6.0	1.5	46	270	3	410
rigatoni in cream sauce w/broccoli & chicken	1 entree	6.0	2.0	40	260	2	480
spaghetti marinara, low fat	1 entree	6.0	1.5	45	270	3	680
ziti Parmesano, low fat	1 entrée	7.0	2.0	42	260	3	530
Weight Watchers Smart Ones							
lasagna Bolognese	1 entree	3.0	1.0	43	240	4	560
macaroni & beef in tomato sauce	1 entree	5.0	2.0	45	280	7	490
ravioli Florentine	1 entree	5.0	2.0	34	220	3	510
three-cheese ziti marinara	1 entree	7.0	2.0	47	290	5	600
Mexican Dinners and Entrees							
Amy's Kitchen							
bean & cheese burrito	1 each	8.0	2.5	43	280	6	540
black bean enchilada	1 meal	8.0	1.0	55	320	9	740
black bean vegetable burrito	1 each	8.0	1.0	44	280	4	580
Burrito Especial	1 each	6.0	1.5	45	260	3	620
Mexican tamale pie	1 each						
Santa Fe enchilada bowl	1 bowl	9.0	2.0	47	340	10	780
Café Classics, Lean Cuisine							
Fiesta grilled chicken	1 meal	6.0	2.5	31	260	3	580
Everyday Foods, Lean Cuisine							
chicken enchilada	1 meal	5.0	2.0	48	290	3	560

	Serving	Total Fat (g)	Saturated Fat (g)	Total Carbohydrate (g)	Total Calories	Dietary Fiber	Sodium (mg)
Santa Fe rice & beans	1 meal	5.0	2.0	53	300	5	580
three-bean chili	1 entree	7.0	2.0	43	270	8	630
Healthy Choice, chicken enchiladas	1 meal	7.0	3.0	59	360	8	580
Healthy Choice Solos, chicken enchilada	1 meal	7.0	2.5	48	300	6	600
Ortega							
chicken fajita skillet	8 oz.	4.0	2.0	12	140	4	515
steak fajita skillet	8 oz.	4.0	2.0	12	140	4	764
Patio							
bean & cheese burrito	1 each	9.0	4.5	46	300	4	690
beef & bean burrito	1 each	10.0	5.0	45	310	4	860
chicken burrito	1 each	8.0	3.0	44	290	2	740
enchilada, beef	2 pieces	8.0	3.0	29	210	5	940
enchilada, cheese	2 pieces	7.0	3.5	30	210	2	880
Tyson Meal Kits							
beef fajitas	2 fajitas	10.0	3.0	42	320	4	740
chicken fajitas	2 fajitas	7.0	2.0	34	260	4	700
chicken quesadillas	1 each	10.0	5.0	26	250	3	430
Weight Watchers							
chicken enchilada suiza	1 each	10.0	4.0	33	283	4	520
Pizza, frozen varieties							
Amy's Kitchen pizza							
cheese	1 pizza	12.0	4.0	38	300	2	540
mushroom & olive	1 pizza	9.0	3.0	33	250	2	560
pesto	1 pizza	12.0	3.5	39	310	2	480
roasted vegetable	1 pizza	8.0	1.5	42	260	2	490
soy cheese	1 pizza	11.0	1.0	37	290	2	590
spinach	1 pizza	12.0	4.0	38	300	2	590
veggie combo	1 pizza	11.0	3.0	36	290	1	580
Amy's Kitchen pizza snack bites							
cheese	6 pieces	6.0	3.0	22	180	2	290
spinach & feta	6 pieces	6.0	3.0	24	170	2	430
Banquet snack style cheese pizza	6 pieces	8.0	4.0	24	200	2	360
Boca Foods vegetarian pizza							
pepperoni, tomato, & herb	1/3 whole	8.0	3.5	30	240	4	670
supreme	1/3 whole	8.0	3.5	30	250	3	750

	Serving	Total Fat (g)	Saturated Fat (g)	Total Carbohydrate (g)	Total Calories	Dietary Fiber	Sodium (mg)
Café Classics pizzas, Lean Cuisine							
deluxe	1 6-oz. pizza	9.0	3.5	55	370	3	590
four cheese	1 6-oz. pizza	7.0	3.0	60	380	3	690
pepperoni	1 6-oz. pizza	9.0	4.0	57	380	3	680
roasted vegetable	1 6-oz. pizza	4.5	1.5	35	330	3	560
DiGiorno rising-crust pizza							
chicken supreme	1 piece	9.0	4.5	33	270	2	740
four cheese	1 piece	11.0	6.0	39	320	3	870
spinach	1 piece	8.0	4.0	33	250	3	670
vegetable	1 piece	10.0	5.0	41	310	3	830
Healthy Choice French bread pizza							
cheese	1 pizza	5.0	1.5	57	360	5	600
pepperoni	1 pizza	5.0	1.5	56	360	6	600
supreme	1 pizza	5.0	1.5	58	360	8	600
vegetable	1 pizza	5.0	1.5	50	320	4	600
Jack's pizza							
Canadian bacon, naturally rising	1 piece	9.0	5.0	34	280	2	590
Canadian bacon, original	1 piece	10.0	5.0	31	280	2	620
cheese, naturally rising	1 piece	10.0	6.0	35	290	2	500
Kid Cuisine pizza							
Fire Chief cheese	1 pizza	10.0	5.0	44	340	2	780
Pirate cheese pizza dinner	1 meal	11.0	5.0	71	430	5	480
Lean Cuisine French bread pizzas							
cheese	1 pizza	7.0	4.0	47	320	3	520
deluxe	1 pizza	9.0	3.5	44	310	3	700
pepperoni	1 pizza	7.0	2.5	44	300	2	560
Stouffer's French bread grilled vegetable pizza	1 pizza	12.0	5.0	48	350	3	500
Tombstone Pizza for One							
cheese, 1/2 less fat	1 pizza	10.0	4.5	43	380	3	940
vegetable, 1/2 less fat	1 pizza	9.0	4.0	48	360	5	860
Tombstone Supreme light pizza	1 piece	9.0	3.5	30	270	3	720
Totino's pizza							
microwave cheese pizza for one	1 pizza	11.0	3.5	26	240	1	540
Totino's cheese pizza rolls	6 each	8.0	2.5	25	210	1	420

	Serving	Total Fat (g)	Saturated Fat (g)	Total Carbohydrate (g)	Total Calories	Dietary Fiber	Sodium (mg)
Sandwiches, frozen varieties							
Amy's Kitchen in-a-pocket-sandwiches							
broccoli & cheese	1 each	10.0	4.0	37	270	3	560
cheese pizza	1 each	9.0	3.5	42	300	4	450
roasted vegetables	1 each	8.0	1.5	35	220	4	480
soy cheese pizza	1 each	8.0	0.5	39	260	6	520
spinach feta	1 each	9.0	4.5	34	250	3	590
tofu scramble	1 each	6.0	0.0	23	180	1	520
vegetable pie	1 each	9.0	1.5	45	300	3	490
vegetarian pizza	1 each	6.0	2.5	39	250	4	360
Banquet sandwich toppings							
beef, creamed chipped	4 oz.	6.0	2.5	8	120	0	700
beef, sliced, w/gravy	4 oz.	2.0	1.0	5	70	0	440
Healthy Choice sandwiches							
chicken & broccoli	1 each	4.0	1.5	50	310	2	600
ham & cheese	1 each	5.0	1.5	48	320	1	590
meatball, Italian style	1 each	5.0	1.5	52	330	4	600
Philly beef steak	1 each	5.0	1.5	50	310	3	600
Lean Pockets							
bacon, egg, & cheese	1 each	4.5	1.0	45	150	2	280
barbecue	1 each	7.0	2.0	47	290	3	850
cheeseburger	1 each	7.0	3.0	42	280	4	810
chicken, cheddar, & broccoli	1 each	7.0	2.0	39	260	3	590
chicken fajita	1 each	7.0	2.5	38	260	3	730
chicken parmesan	1 each	7.0	2.5	43	280	3	620
ham & cheddar	1 each	7.0	2.5	40	280	3	700
meatballs & mozzarella	1 each	7.0	2.5	44	290	3	700
pepperoni pizza	1 each	7.0	2.5	42	280	4	720
Philly steak & cheese	1 each	7.0	2.5	40	280	3	590
sausage & pepperoni pizza	1 each	7.0	2.5	41	280	4	630
sausage, egg, & cheese	1 each	4.5	1.5	19	140	2	310
steak fajita	1 each	7.0	2.0	39	260	3	730
turkey & ham w/cheddar	1 each	7.0	2.0	43	280	3	710
turkey, broccoli, & cheese	1 each	7.0	2.5	39	270	3	530
Morningstar Farms vegetarian sandwiches							
English muffin w/egg & patty	1 each	2.5	0.0	34	240	3	390

	Serving	Total Fat (g)	Saturated Fat (g)	Total Carbohydrate (g)	Total Calories	Dietary Fiber	Sodium (mg)
English muffin w/egg, patty, & cheese	1 each	3.0	0.0	33	280	7	1000
stuffed burger & cheese	1 each	8.0	3.5	40	290	2	390
stuffed ham & cheese	1 each	7.0	3.0	45	301	2	520
stuffed pepperoni pizza	1 each	7.0	3.0	42	280	5	420
Ore-Ida chicken fajita sandwich	1 each	8.0	2.0	35	250	3	390
Weight Watchers On-the-Go chicken, broccoli, & cheddar pocket	1 each	6.0	2.0	40	265	3	390
Vegetarian/Meatless Meals and Entrees							
Amy's Kitchen							
All-American burger	1 each	3.0	0.0	15	120	3	390
California burger	1 each	5.0	0.5	19	130	5	430
Chicago burger	1 each	5.0	1.5	20	160	3	390
Texas burger	1 each	2.5	0.0	14	120	3	350
Boca Foods							
All-American flame-grilled burger	1 each	4.0	1.0	5	110	3	360
cheeseburger	1 each						
grilled veggie burger	1 each	1.0	0.0	6	80	4	320
ground burger	1/2 cup	0.5	0.0	7	70	4	220
Original burger	1 each	1.0	0.0	6	80	4	320
Original chik'n nuggets							
Original or spicy chik'n patties	1 each	6.0	0.5	11	160	2	430
roasted garlic burger	1 each	1.5	0.0	6	90	4	440
roasted onion burger	1 each	1.0	0.0	7	80	4	300
Cedarlane							
Mediterranean stuffed focaccia	1/3 focaccia	10.0	6.0	37	296	1	485
Roma tomato & basil stuffed focaccia	1/3 focaccia	9.0	4.0	33	275	2	528
veggie "pepperoni" stuffed focaccia	1/3 focaccia	6.0	4.0	34	250	1	430
Morningstar Farms							
buffalo wings	5 wings	9.0	1.5	18	200	6	630
Chik Patties chicken substitute	1 patty	6.0	1.0	16	150	2	540

	Serving	Total Fat (g)	Saturated Fat (g)	Total Carbohydrate (g)	Total Calories	Dietary Fiber	Sodium (mg)
Chik Patties Parmesan ranch	1 patty	7.0	1.0	17	170	2	680
chili pot pie	1 each	9.0	1.0	49	330	7	870
corn dogs	1 each	4.0	0.5	22	150	3	500
veggie burgers							
Better'N Burgers veggie burger	1 each	2.0	0.0	6	100	3	310
fajita burgers	1 each	7.0	2.0	7	130	3	290
Garden Veggie burger	1 each	2.5	0.5	9	100	4	350
Griller's Original veggie burger	1 each	6.0	1.0	5	140	2	260
Griller's Prime veggie burger	1 each	9.0	1.0	5	170	2	390
Harvest burger	1 each	4.0	1.5	8	140	5	390
Philly cheese steak burger	1 each	6.0	1.5	6	120	3	400
portobello mushrooms & roasted peppers veggie burger	1 each	4.0	0.5	9	120	3	470
spicy black bean burger	1 each	4.5	0.5	16	150	5	470
tomato & basil pizza burger	1 each	6.0	1.5	7	130	3	320
Natural Touch							
classic burger	1 each	7.0	1.0	10	150	3	340
lentil rice loaf	1 slice	7.0	1.0	16	160	4	350
nine-bean loaf	1 slice	7.0	1.5	15	150	4	320
roasted herb chik'n	1 patty	2.5	0.5	9	110	2	380
vegetarian chili	1 cup	1.0	0.0	21	170	11	870
vegetarian tuno tuna fish substitute	1/3 cup	2.0	0.5	2	60	1	360
veggie corn dogs	1 each	6.0	1.0	22	170	3	530
zesty tomato basil burger	1 each	6.0	1.0	7	130	4	290

Frozen Foods/Potatoes and Side Dishes

Criterion for general selection: ≤ 3 grams fat per serving (1/2 cup)

Potatoes

	Serving	Total Fat (g)	Saturated Fat (g)	Total Carbohydrate (g)	Total Calories	Dietary Fiber	Sodium (mg)
Bird's Eye							
baby gourmet	7 (4 oz.)	0.0	0.0	21	100	1	15
whole	3 (2.6 oz.)	0.0	0.0	15	50	1	25
Everyday Foods, Lean Cuisine							
roasted potatoes w/broccoli	1 cup	5.0	3.0	37	240	4	660
Fit Fries, entree cut	3 oz.	2.5	0.5	20	110	3	55
Green Giant							
potatoes w/broccoli in cheese sauce	3/4 cup	3.5	1.5	19	120	2	520

	Serving	Total Fat (g)	Saturated Fat (g)	Total Carbohydrate (g)	Total Calories	Dietary Fiber	Sodium (mg)
Healthy Choice							
cheddar broccoli potatoes	1 meal	7.0	3.0	41	270	7	600
MicroMagic french fries, low fat	1 pkg.	3.0	1.0	23	130	3	35
Ore-Ida							
Golden Fries	3 oz.	3.5	1.0	20	120	2	360
hashbrowns, country, or Southern style	1/2 cup	0.0	0.0	12	60	2	15
mashed w/natural butter flavor	1/2 cup	2.0	0.5	14	80	1	140
O'Brien	1/2 cup	0.0	0.0	12	55	2	15
wedges w/skin, homestyle	1 each	2.3	0.9	17	100	2	15
Side Dishes (Vegetables and/or Pasta or Rice)							
Bird's Eye International Recipes							
Bavarian style w/noodles	1/2 cup	2.7	1.5	6	55	1	150
Italian style green beans w/egg noodles	1/2 cup	3.1	1.2	5	50	1	130
Green Giant							
broccoli, carrots, & liflower skillet	2/3 cup	0.0	0.0	4	25	2	30 cau-
broccoli, carrots, & water chestnuts stir fry	2/3 cup	0.0	0.0	5	25	2	30
broccoli, cauliflower, & carrots w/butter sauce	3/4 cup	2.0	1.5	8	60	2	300
broccoli, cauliflower, & carrots w/cheese sauce	2/3 cup	2.5	1.5	11	80	2	560
broccoli w/cheese sauce	1 cup	4.2	0.8	15	110	3	805
Brussels sprouts w/butter sauce	2/3 cup	1.5	1.0	9	60	4	270
carrots, honey glazed	1 cup	3.5	0.5	13	90	2	140
corn, Niblets, w/butter sauce	2/3 cup	3.0	1.5	23	130		350
corn, southwestern style	3/4 cup	1.0	0.0	18	90	1	130
corn, white, shoepeg, w/butter sauce	3/4 cup	2.5	1.5	21	120	3	320
mixed vegetables w/butter sauce	3/4 cup	2.0	1.0	11	75	3	250
peas, early w/butter sauce	3/4 cup	2.0	1.5	16	100	4	370
peas, sweet w/butter sauce	3/4 cup	2.0	1.5	15	100	5	400

	Serving	Total Fat (g)	Saturated Fat (g)	Total Carbohydrate (g)	Total Calories	Dietary Fiber	Sodium (mg)
spinach, creamed	½ cup	3.0	1.5	10	80	2	520
spinach, leaf, cut w/butter sauce	½ cup	1.5	1.0	5	40	2	280
vegetables, Alfredo w/cream sauce	¾ cup	3.0	1.5	9	80	3	450
Green Giant Pasta Accents							
pasta w/vegetables							
Alfredo	½ cup	2.0	0.6	6	50	1	120
creamy cheddar	½ cup	1.7	0.6	8	55	1	150
Florentine	½ cup	2.3	0.8	11	80	1	230
garden herb seasoning	½ cup	1.8	1.0	8	60	2	190
garlic seasoning	½ cup	2.5	1.3	9	65	1	160
Oriental style	½ cup	2.0	0.8	7	50	1	115
primavera	½ cup	2.0	0.6	9	65	1	12
white cheddar sauce	½ cup	2.5	0.7	11	80	1	215
Green Giant Rice and Vegetable Combos							
rice pilaf w/vegetables	1 each	3.0	1.5	44	230	3	1020
rice w/vegetable medley	1 each	3.0	1.5	46	240	3	880

Frozen Foods/Desserts

Criterion for general selection: ≤ 4 grams fat per serving (½ cup or 2-ounce slice)

Ice Milk, Frozen Yogurt, Sherbets, Dessert Bars, Popsicles

	Serving	Total Fat (g)	Saturated Fat (g)	Total Carbohydrate (g)	Total Calories	Dietary Fiber	Sodium (mg)
Breyers							
All Natural Light varieties							
French vanilla	½ cup	4.0	2.0	18	120	0	50
natural vanilla	½ cup	3.0	2.0	17	110	0	50
98% fat-free chocolate or vanilla	½ cup	1.5	1.0	21	90	4	50
98% fat-free frozen yogurt	½ cup	1.5	1.0	23	120	0	55
vanilla/chocolate/ strawberry	½ cup	3.0	2.0	18	110	0	45
no sugar added varieties							
chocolate caramel	½ cup	4.0	2.5	18	110	<1	55
chocolate fudge brownie	½ cup	1.5	1.0	20	90	4	85
vanilla/chocolate/ strawberry	½ cup	4.0	2.5	15	100	0	50
vanilla fudge twirl	½ cup	4.0	2.5	19	110	<1	50
sherbet, orange or rainbow	½ cup	1.5	1.0	27	130	0	25

	Serving	Total Fat (g)	Saturated Fat (g)	Total Carbohydrate (g)	Total Calories	Dietary Fiber	Sodium (mg)
Dole Fruit 'n Juice bars, all flavors, avg.	1 each	0.0	0.0	18	70	0	5
Edy's							
frozen yogurt varieties							
Chocolate Decadence	1/2 cup	3.5	1.5	20	120	0	45
Cookies 'N Cream	1/2 cup	3.5	1.5	19	120	0	45
HEATH Toffee Crunch	1/2 cup	4.0	2.0	18	120	0	45
raspberry	1/2 cup	2.5	1.5	16	90	0	25
vanilla	1/2 cup	2.5	1.5	17	100	0	30
frozen yogurt, fat-free varieties							
Black Cherry Vanilla Swirl	1/2 cup	0.0	0.0	20	90	0	45
Caramel Praline Crunch	1/2 cup	0.0	0.0	23	100	0	60
Coffee Fudge Sundae	1/2 cup	0.0	0.0	22	100	0	60
vanilla or vanilla chocolate swirl	1/2 cup	0.0	0.0	19	90	0	45
Grand Light varieties							
chocolate	1/2 cup	3.5	2.0	16	110	0	45
Cookies 'n Cream	1/2 cup	4.0	2.0	18	120	0	60
French vanilla	1/2 cup	3.5	2.0	15	120	0	45
Fudge Tracks	1/2 cup	4.0	2.5	18	120	0	50
Neopolitan	1/2 cup	3.0	2.0	15	100	0	40
Rocky Road	1/2 cup	4.0	2.0	17	120	0	40
strawberry	1/2 cup	2.5	1.5	17	100	0	40
vanilla	1/2 cup	3.5	2.0	15	100	0	45
no-sugar-added varieties							
chocolate	1/2 cup	3.0	1.5	13	90	0	45
Cookie Dough	1/2 cup	4.0	2.5	16	110	0	65
Double Fudge Brownie	1/2 cup	3.5	2.0	17	110	0	55
Mint Chocolate Chips!	1/2 cup	3.0	1.5	13	90	0	50
Neopolitan	1/2 cup	3.0	1.5	13	90	0	50
strawberry	1/2 cup	3.0	1.5	13	90	0	50
Triple Chocolate	1/2 cup	3.0	2.0	16	100	0	55
vanilla	1/2 cup	3.0	1.5	14	100	0	50
no-sugar-added fat-free varieties							
chocolate fudge	1/2 cup	0.0	0.0	22	100	0	60
raspberry vanilla swirl	1/2 cup	0.0	0.0	19	90	0	50
vanilla	1/2 cup	0.0	0.0	20	90	0	50
vanilla chocolate swirl	1/2 cup	0.0	0.0	20	100	0	50

	Serving	Total Fat (g)	Saturated Fat (g)	Total Carbohydrate (g)	Total Calories	Dietary Fiber	Sodium (mg)
Fudgsicle							
fat-free	1 each	0.0	0.0	15	60	0	50
pops	1 each	1.0	0.0	26	120	0	75
sugar free	1 each	0.5	0.0	9	40	0	35
Häagen-Dazs							
bars							
chocolate sorbet	1 each	0.0	0.0	20	80	1	50
raspberry sorbet w/vanilla yogurt	1 each	0.0	0.0	21	90	<1	12
frozen yogurt							
Chocolate Fudge Brownie	1/2 cup	2.5	1.5	35	200	2	140
Dulce de Leche	1/2 cup	2.5	2.0	35	190	0	75
strawberry banana	1/2 cup	2.0	1.0	30	160	<1	25
strawberry, fat-free	1/2 cup	0.0	0.0	31	140	0	40
vanilla raspberry swirl	1/2 cup	2.5	1.5	31	170	<1	30
sorbets							
chocolate	1/2 cup	0.5	0.0	28	130	2	70
mango	1/2 cup	0.0	0.0	31	120	<1	0
orange	1/2 cup	0.0	0.0	30	120	<1	0
Orchard Peach	1/2 cup	0.0	0.0	33	130	<1	0
raspberry	1/2 cup	0.0	0.0	30	120	2	0
strawberry	1/2 cup	0.0	0.0	30	120	1	0
Zesty Lemon	1/2 cup	0.0	0.0	31	120	<1	0
Healthy Choice ice creams							
Brownie Bliss	1/2 cup	2.0	1.0	24	130	1	70
Butter Pecan Crunch	1/2 cup	2.0	1.0	18	100	2	65
Cappuccino Chocolate Chunk	1/2 cup	2.0	1.0	20	120	<1	70
Caramel Fudge Brownie	1/2 cup	2.0	1.0	21	120	1	70
Cherry Chocolate Mambo	1/2 cup	2.0	1.0	23	130	1	70
Chocolate Chocolate Chunk	1/2 cup	2.0	1.0	21	120	1	60
Cookies 'N Cream	1/2 cup	2.0	1.0	21	120	<1	90
Crazy Caramel	1/2 cup	2.0	1.0	23	120	<1	70
Double Karma	1/2 cup	2.0	1.0	28	140	<1	90
French Silk	1/2 cup	1.5	1.0	24	120	2	50
Happy Together	1/2 cup	2.0	1.0	29	150	1	70
Jumpin' Java	1/2 cup	2.0	1.0	25	130	<1	75
Mint Chocolate Chip	1/2 cup	2.0	1.0	20	120	<1	70

	Serving	Total Fat (g)	Saturated Fat (g)	Total Carbohydrate (g)	Total Calories	Dietary Fiber	Sodium (mg)
No Sugar Added Chocolate Fudge Brownie	½ cup	2.0	1.0	21	120	1	60
No Sugar Added Coffee Almond Fudge	½ cup	2.0	1.0	20	110	1	55
No Sugar Added Mint Chocolate Chip	½ cup	2.0	1.0	18	110	1	50
No Sugar Added Vanilla	½ cup	2.0	1.0	17	100	1	55
Peanut Butter Cup	½ cup	2.0	1.0	21	120	<1	70
Praline & Caramel	½ cup	2.0	1.0	23	120	<1	80
Rocky Road	½ cup	2.0	1.0	25	130	<1	60
Tin Roof Sundae	½ cup	2.0	1.0	21	120	1	60
Turtle Fudge Cake	½ cup	2.0	1.0	23	130	<1	70
Vanilla	½ cup	2.0	1.0	19	110	<1	60
Vanilla Bean	½ cup	2.0	1.0	21	120	<1	60
Vanilla Caramel Fudge	½ cup	2.0	1.0	28	140	<1	90
ice cream sandwiches							
Caramel Swirl sandwich	1 each	3.0	1.0	27	140	<1	120
Fudge Swirl sandwich	1 each	3.0	1.0	27	140	<1	150
vanilla sandwich	1 each	3.0	1.0	24	130	<1	150
premium low-fat ice cream bars							
fudge (12 pack)	1 bar	1.5	1.0	15	90	0	70
fudge (6 pack)	1 bar	1.0	0.5	13	80	0	60
mocha fudge swirl (6 pack)	1 bar	1.5	1.0	17	90	1	50
strawberry & cream (12 pack)	1 bar	1.5	1.0	20	110	<1	55
strawberry & cream (6 pack)	1 bar	1.5	1.0	17	90	<1	45
Klondike Slim-A-Bear							
98% fat-free chocolate or vanilla sandwich	1 each	1.5	0.0	28	130	3	120
98% fat-free mint or vanilla sandwich	1 each	1.5	0.0	28	130	3	120
no sugar added vanilla sandwich	1 each	3.0	0.5	25	120	2	230
premium fudge bar	1 each	1.5	0.5	22	90	4	90
Popsicle, all flavors	1 each	0.0	0.0	11	45	0	0
Popsicle sugar-free, all flavors	1 each	0.0	0.0	4	15	0	0

	Serving	Total Fat (g)	Saturated Fat (g)	Total Carbohydrate (g)	Total Calories	Dietary Fiber	Sodium (mg)
Skinny Cow low-fat ice cream sandwiches							
caramel	1 each	2.5	1.0	27	140	2	200
chocolate peanut butter	1 each	2.5	1.0	27	140	2	200
coffee or strawberry shortcake	1 each	2.0	1.0	23	130	2	200
combo or mint or vanilla	1 each	2.0	1.0	23	130	2	200
Welch's fruit juice bars	1 each	0.0	0.0	11	45	0	0
Cakes, Pies							
Chez De Prez cheesecakes, fat-free	2-oz. slice	0.0	0.0	19	90	1	15
Krusteaz cheesecake	2-oz. slice	0.1	0.0	20	100	1	180
Pepperidge Farm apple spice, Dessert Light	4-oz. slice	2.0	0.0	37	170	0	105
Sara Lee							
carrot cake, Lights	2.5-oz. slice	4.0	1.0	30	170	0	75
cheesecake, French, Lights	3-oz. slice	4.0	1.0	24	150	0	90
Free & Light pound cake	1/10 cake	0.0	0.0	17	70	0	105
Weight Watchers							
Boston Cream pie	1/2 pkg.	4.0	1.0	34	160	0	260
brownie à la mode	1 each	4.0	1.0	34	190	2	170
chocolate brownie, frosted	1 each	2.5	1.0	22	100	3	135
chocolate éclair	1 each	4.0	0.7	24	140	1	185
chocolate mocha pie	1 each	4.0	1.0	31	170	2	125
devil's food, Sweet Rewards	1 each	1.5	0.5	36	160	1	370
strawberry cheesecake, Sweet Celebrations	1 each	4.0	1.0	28	180	0	210
triple chocolate cheesecake, Sweet Celebrations	1 each	4.0	1.0	30	190	0	220

Miscellaneous/Jellies, Jams, Syrups, Pickles, Hot Cocoa Mixes
Criteria for general selection: 0 gram fat per serving for jellies, jams, syrups, pickles;
≤ 1 gram fat per 8-ounce (1 cup) serving for hot cocoa
Jellies/Jams (NOTE: all brands meet criteria)
Syrups (NOTE: all brands meet criteria)
Pickles (NOTE: all brands meet criteria)
Hot Cocoa Mixes (1 pkt. = 1 cup prepared)
Criterion for general selection: ≤ 1 gram of fat per cup (8 ounces)

	Serving	Total Fat (g)	Saturated Fat (g)	Total Carbohydrate (g)	Total Calories	Dietary Fiber	Sodium (mg)
Carnation							
double chocolate Meltdown	1 pkt.	3.0	2.5	29	150	1	150
Homemade Classics dark chocolate	1 pkt.	1.1	0.0	22	96	2	75
Homemade Classics milk chocolate	1 pkt.	0.5	0.0	25	96	1	58
rich chocolate, fat-free	1 pkt.	0.0	0.0	4	25	1	130
rich chocolate, fat-free w/marshmallows	1 pkt.	0.0	0.0	8	40	1	125
rich chocolate, sugar-free	1 pkt.	0.5	0.0	9	50	1	170
Swiss Miss							
sugar-free	1 pkt.	1.0	0.0	10	50	1	190
w/marshmallows, w/o added sugar	1 pkt.	1.0	0.0	10	60	1	180
Vita soy light cocoa	1 pkt.	2.0	0.0	25	130	2	130

APPENDIX A

CHOLESTEROL CONTENT OF COMMON FOODS

Dietary cholesterol is a fatlike substance found only in foods of animal origin. Plant foods do not contain cholesterol. Dietary cholesterol is highest in organ meats and found in varying amounts in other meats, poultry, fish, shellfish, dairy foods, and animal fats. Your *blood* cholesterol level is affected by the types of fats in your diet (a diet high in saturated fat raises blood cholesterol) more so than by the cholesterol you eat in food. The American Heart Association recommends consuming less than 300 milligrams (mg.) of cholesterol a day on average. The following list provides the cholesterol content of common foods—you can also find the cholesterol content of the foods you buy by checking the food labels.

Food	Cholesterol mg.
Beef/Pork (averages)	
bacon, 3 strips, cooked, 1 oz.	20
fattier cuts, cooked, 3 oz.	100
ground beef, lean, 3 oz.	75
hot dog, 1	29
lean cuts, cooked, 3 oz.	70
Chicken/Turkey (averages)	
dark meat, cooked, 3 oz.	90
white meat, cooked, 3 oz.	70
Organ Meats	
beef/calf liver, braised, 3 oz.	400
brains, beef, fried, 3 oz.	1,400
chicken liver, 3oz.	540
Fish and Shellfish	
flounder/haddock/sole, baked, 3 oz.	70
salmon, broiled, 3 oz.	40
shrimp, large, boiled, 8	87
tuna, canned in water, 3 oz.	30
Egg, large, cooked	
white	0
yolk	213
Dairy Foods	
cheese, American, 1 oz.	27
cheese, cheddar, 1 oz.	30
cheese, mozzarella, part skim, 1 oz.	16
cheese, low-fat varieties, 1 oz.	7

cottage cheese, creamed, 4% fat, $^1/_2$ cup	16
cottage cheese, 1% low fat, $^1/_2$ cup	5
cream, $^1/_2$ & $^1/_2$, 1 T.	10
cream, sour, 1 T.	6
cream cheese, 1 T.	16
ice milk or frozen yogurt, $^1/_2$ cup	10
ice cream, 10% fat, $^1/_2$ cup	30
nonfat/skim milk, 1 cup	4
pudding, w/2% milk, $^1/_2$ cup	10
1% milk, 1 cup	10
2% milk, 1 cup	22
whole milk, 1 cup	34
yogurt, nonfat, 1 cup	10
yogurt, whole milk, 1 cup	29

Fats
butter, 1 t.	11
margarine, 1 t.	0
mayonnaise, 1 T.	10
mayonnaise, reduced fat, 1 T.	5

Other Foods (averages)
brownie, chocolate, 2 × 2″	15
cake, yellow w/frosting, $^1/_{12}$ cake	55
candy bar, chocolate, 1 oz.	4
cheesecake, traditional, $^1/_8$ pie	45
chili w/beans, 1 cup	50
cookie, chocolate chip, homemade	10
cream soup, made w/2% milk, 1 cup	12
egg roll, 1 restaurant style	50
fettuccine Alfredo, 1 cup	75
lasagna, w/meat & cheese, 1 cup	80
pizza, cheese, $^1/_8$ large	40
pizza, combination w/meat, $^1/_8$ large	60
soup, beef w/noodles or vegetables, 1 cup	15
soup, chicken w/noodles or vegetables, 1 cup	15
soup, cream, reconstituted w/water, 1 cup	20
spaghetti w/meat sauce, 1 cup	56
sushi w/fish & vegetables, 5 oz.	10
taco, hard shell w/meat & cheese	55

APPENDIX B

FOOD COMPANY WEB SITES

Here are the World Wide Web sites for literally hundreds of food companies organized by parent companies with their subsidiaries or brand Web sites. The majority of these Web sites include nutrition information for their brand-specific food products. As food companies add, remove, or reformulate food products frequently, these Web sites may provide a way to check or verify nutrition information on the brands you buy. Parent companies are listed alphabetically with Web sites for their subsidiary brands. Also, look for Web-site addresses on the food labels of the foods you buy.

Parent Company	Subsidiary Brand-Name Web Sites
American Pop Corn Company	www.JollyTime.com
Amy's Kitchen, Inc.	www.Amys.com
Archway Cookies, LLC	www.ArchwayCookies.com
Authentic Foods Company	www.Gardenburger.com
Azteca Foods, Inc.	www.AztecaFoods.com
B & G Foods, Inc.	www.BGFoods.com
	www.Ortega.com
	www.RedDevilSauce.com
The B. Manischewitz Company, LLC	www.Manischewitz.com
Barbara's Bakery	www.BarbarasBakery.com
Bird's Eye Foods, Inc.	www.BirdseyeFoods.com
Bob Evans Farms, Inc.	www.BobEvans.com
Bob's Red Mill Natural Foods	www.BobsRedMill.com
Bush Brothers & Company	www.BushBeans.com
Cadbury Schweppes PLC	www.CadburySchweppes.com
Cadbury	www.Cadbury.co.uk
Dr Pepper/7Up, Inc.	www.DPSU.com
Mott's Inc.	www.Motts.com
	www.Clamato.com
	www.GrandmaMolasses.com
	www.MottsProducts.com
	www.ReaLemon.com
Snapple Beverage Corporation	www.Snapple.com
California Sun Dry	www.CalSunDry.com
Campbell Soup Company	www.CampbellSoup.com
	www.Godiva.com
	www.PaceFoods.com

	www.PFGoldFish.com
	www.PuffPastry.com
	www.Spaghettios.com
	www.SwansonBroth.com
	www.v8Juice.com
Carl Buddig & Company	www.Buddig.com
Chattanooga Bakeries	www.MoonPie.com
Chef Paul Prudhomme	www.ChefPaul.com
Chelsea Milling Company	www.JiffyMix.com
Chicken of the Sea International	www.ChickenOfTheSea.com
Chiquita Brands, Inc.	www.Chiquita.com
Clif Bar Inc.	www.ClifBar.com
The Coca-Cola Company	www.CocaCola.com
	www.MinuteMaid.com
	www.Powerade.com
	www.SimplyOrangeJuice.com
ConAgra Foods, Inc	www.ConAgraFoods.com
	www.ActII.com
	www.BlueBonnet.com
	www.Butterball.com
	www.ChefBoyardee.com
	www.CooksHam.com
	www.EckrichBrand.com
	www.EggBeaters.com
	www.Fleischmanns.com
	www.HealthyChoice.com
	www.HebrewNational.com
	www.Hunts.com
	www.HuntsSnackPack.com
	www.LifeChoice.com
	www.LightLife.com
	www.Orville.com
	www.Pam4You.com
	www.Parkay.com
	www.Reddi-Wip.com
	www.Ro-Tel.com
	www.SlimJim.com
	www.WolfBrandChili.com
	www.WolfgangPuck.com
Bumble Bee Seafoods, LLC	www.BumbleBee.com
Lamb-Weston, Inc.	www.Lamb-Weston.com
Louis Kemp Seafood Company	www.LouisKemp.com

Continental Mills, Inc.	www.ContinentalMills.com
	www.EagleMills.com
	www.Ghirardelli.com
	www.SunMaid.com
CoolBrands International, Inc.	www.EskimoPie.com
	www.FruitAFreeze.com
Dean Foods	www.DeanFoods.com
	www.BerkeleyFarms.com
	www.FolgersJakada.com
	www.HorizonOrganic.com
	www.InternationalDelight.com
	www.Maries.com
	www.MayfieldDairy.com
WhiteWave	www.WhiteWave.com
Silk	www.SilkisSoy.com
SunSoy	www.SunSoy.com
Del Monte Foods	www.DelMonte.com
	www.CollegeInn.com
	www.Contadina.com
	www.NaturesGoodness.com
	www.Starkist.com
	www.SWFineFoods.com
Dole Food Company, Inc.	www.Dole.com
Dryers, Inc.	www.DryersInc.com
Dreyer's Grand Ice Cream	www.Dreyers.com
Edy's Grand Ice Cream	www.Edys.com
	www.NestleIceCream.com
Eagle Family Foods, Inc.	www.EagleBrand.com
Fantastic Foods	www.FantasticFoods.com
General Mills, Inc.	www.GeneralMills.com
	www.BettyCrocker.com
	www.Bugles.com
	www.HaagenDazs.com
	www.LloydsBBQ.com
	www.MuirGlen.com
	www.NatureValley.com
	www.PopSecret.com
	www.ProgressoSoup.com
	www.YoplaitUSA.com
The Pillsbury Company	www.Pillsbury.com
	www.GreenGiant.com
	www.OldElPaso.com

Small Planet Foods	www.SmallPlanetFoods.com
	www.CascadianFarms.com
	www.MuirGlenOrganic.com
Geni-Soy	www.GeniSoy.com
George Weston Bakeries, Inc.	www.GWBakeries.com
	www.Boboli.com
Gerber	www.Gerber.com
Ghiradelli	www.Ghiradelli.com
Godiva	www.Godiva.com
Golden Grain Company	www.Goldengrain-Mission.com
Gorton's	www.Gortons.com
Goya Foods, Inc.	www.GoyaFoods.com
Groupe DANONE	www.DanoneGroup.com
The Dannon Company, Inc.	www.Dannon.com
Evian	www.Evian.com
Häagen-Dazs	www.Haagen-Dazs.com
The Hain Celestial Group, Inc.	www.Hain-Celestial.com
	www.Alba.com
	www.ArrowHeadMills.com
	www.CarbFit.com
	www.CelestialSeasonings.com
	www.EarthsBest.com
	www.EsteeFoods.com
	www.GardenOfEatin.com
	www.HainPureFoods.com
	www.HealthValley.com
	www.ImagineFoods.com
	www.TerraChips.com
	www.Westbrae.com
	www.WestSoy.biz
	www.YvesVeggie.com
Hershey Foods Corporation	www.Hersheys.com
H. J. Heinz Company	www.Heinz.com
	www.BagelBites.com
	www.Orelda.com
Hidden Valley	www.HiddenValley.com
Hodgson Mills, Inc.	www.HodgsonMill.com
Hormel Foods Corporation	www.Hormel.com
	www.AlwaysTender.com
	www.CarapelliUSA.com
	www.ChiChiSalsa.com

	www.DiamondCrystal.com
	www.DintyMoore.com
	www.HormelPepperoni.com
	www.Spam.com
	www.StaggChili.com
Jennie-O Foods, Inc.	www.Jennie-OTurkeyStore.com
Interstate Bakeries Corporation	www.InterstateBakeriesCorp.com
	www.Colombo.com
	www.MarieCalender.com
	www.WonderBread.com
J. M. Smucker's Company	www.Smuckers.com
	www.Crisco.com
	www.HungryJack.com
	www.Jif.com
	www.MarthaWhite.com
	www.PetEvaporatedMilk.com
	www.RobinHood.com
The Kellogg Company	www.KelloggCompany.com
Kashi	www.Kashi.com
Keebler	www.Keebler.com
	www.Cheez-It.com
	www.ReadyCrust.com
Kelloggs	www.Kelloggs.com
Morningstar Farms	www.MorningstarFarms.com
KF Holdings	www.NabiscoWorld.com
Kraft Foods, Inc.	www.KraftFoods.com
	www.A1Marinades.com
	www.Altoids.com
	www.Athenos.com
	www.BakersChocolate.com
	www.Balance.com
	www.BocaBurger.com
	www.Breakstone.com
	www.BreyersYogurt.com
	www.CandyStand.com
	www.CapriSun.com
	www.CoolWhip.com
	www.CornNuts.com
	www.CountryTime.com
	www.CreamofWheat.com
	www.CrystalLight.com

www.DeliDeluxe.com
www.Gevalia.com
www.GFIC.com
www.GoodSeasons.com
www.GreyPoupon.com
www.HandiSnacks.com
www.ItsPastaAnytime.com
www.JacksPizza.com
www.Jello.com
www.JetPuffed.com
www.Knox.com
www.Kool-Aid.com
www.Kraft-Cheese.com
www.KraftEasyMac.com
www.LightNLively.com
www.Lunchables.com
www.MaxwellHouse.com
www.MinuteRice.com
www.MinuteTapioca.com
www.MiracleWhip.com
www.OscarMayer.com
www.Planters.com
www.Polly-O.com
www.StellaDoro.com
www.StoveTop.com
www.TheCheesiest.com
www.Toblerone.com
www.Tombstone.com
www.Velveeta.com
www.Yuban.com
www.Marzetti.com

Lancaster Colony
  Sister Shubert's
Lance, Inc.
Land O' Lakes

Luigino's, Inc.
Malt-O-Meal Company
Mars, Inc.

McKee Foods Corporation

www.SSRolls.com
www.LanceSnacks.com
www.LandOLakes.com
www.AlpineLace.com
www.Michelinas.com
www.Malt-O-Meal.com
www.Mars.com
www.UncleBens.com
www.McKeeFoods.com
www.LittleDebbie.com

	www.SunBeltSnacks.com
Mrs. Smith's Bakeries	www.MrsSmiths.com
Mt. Olive Pickle Company, Inc.	www.MtOlivePickles.com
Nestlé USA, Inc.	www.NestleUSA.com
	www.Buitoni.com
	www.Butterfinger.com
	www.CarnationInstantBreakfast.com
	www.Coffee-Mate.com
	www.HotPockets.com
	www.JuicyJuice.com
	www.LeanCuisine.com
	www.NescafeUSA.com
	www.Nesquik.com
	www.Nestea.com
	www.NestleCrunch.com
	www.NestleHotCocoa.com
	www.NestleSweetTarts.com
	www.OvenSensations.com
	www.PowerBar.com
	www.Stouffers.com
	www.TastersChoice.com
	www.Wonderball.com
	www.Wonka.com
Newman's Own	www.NewmansOwn.com
New World Pasta Company	www.NewWorldPasta.com
	www.AmericanBeauty.com
	www.Creamette.com
	www.LightNFluffy.com
	www.MrsWeiss.com
	www.PrincePasta.com
	www.Ronzoni.com
	www.SanGiorgio.com
NutraSweet Property Holdings, Inc.	www.NutraSweet.com
Ocean Spray Cranberries, Inc	www.OceanSpray.com
Ore-Ida	www.OreIda.com
Otis Spunkmeyer, Inc.	www.Spunkmeyer.com
Pace Foods	www.PaceFoods.com
PepsiCo, Inc.	www.PepsiCo.com
Frito-Lay	www.FritoLay.com
Gatorade	www.Gatorade.com
Quaker Foods	www.QuakerOats.com

	www.AJCornMeal.com
	www.AuntJemima.com
	www.Kretschmer.com
	www.MothersNatural.com
	www.NearEast.com
	www.PastaRoni.com
	www.QuakerChewy.com
	www.QuakerGrits.com
	www.QuakerOatmeal.com
	www.QuakerQuakes.com
	www.Quisp.com
	www.RiceARoni.com
	www.TortillaMix.com
Tropicana	www.Tropicana.com
Perdue Farms, Inc.	www.Perdue.com
Performance Food Group	www.PFG.com
Fresh Express	www.FreshExpress.com
Pinnacle Foods Corporation	www.PinnacleFoodsCorp.com
	www.CelestePizza.com
	www.DuncanHines.com
	www.Swanson.com
	www.Vlasic.com
Procter & Gamble	www.ProcterGamble.com
	www.Folgers.com
	www.Millstone.com
	www.Pringles.com
	www.SunnyD.com
Ralcorp Holdings, Inc.	www.Ralcorp.com
	www.BakeryChef.com
	www.BremmerBiscuit.com
	www.CarriageHouseCos.com
	www.NutcrackerBrands.com
	www.RalstonFoods.com
Rich-SeaPak Corporation	www.Rich-SeaPak.com
	www.ByronsBBQ.com
	www.CasaDiBertacchi.com
	www.FarmRichFun.com
	www.Richs.com
	www.SeaPakShrimp.com
Riviana Foods	www.Riviana.com
	www.CarolinaRice.com

	www.GourmetHouseRice.com
	www.MahatmaRice.com
	www.RiverRice.com
	www.S-and-WRice.com
	www.SuccessRice.com
	www.WaterMaidRice.com
Sara Lee Corporation	www.SaraLee.com
	www.BallPark.com
	www.BryanFoods.com
	www.EarthGrains.com
	www.HillshireFarm.com
	www.IronKids.com
	www.JimmyDean.com
Sargento Foods	www.SargentoCheese.com
Seneca Corporation	www.SenecaFoods.com
Smithfield Foods, Inc.	www.SmithfieldFoods.com
Sunrise Soya Foods	www.Sunrise-Soya.com
	www.PetesTofu.com
Stoneyfield	www.Stoneyfield.com
Sun-Maid	www.Sun-Maid.com
Stadt Corporation	www.SweetOne.com
Sunkist Growers, Inc.	www.Sunkist.com
Swift & Company	www.SwiftBrands.com
Take Control	www.TakeControl.com
Tasty Baking Company	www.TastyKake.com
Tyson Foods	www.Tyson.com
Unilever	www.UnileverNA.com
	www.BenandJerrys.com
	www.Bertolli.com
	www.BestFoods.com
	www.Breyers.com
	www.BrummelandBrown.com
	www.CountryCrock.com
	www.GoodHumor.com
	www.Hellmanns.com
	www.IceCreamUSA.com
	www.Knorr.com
	www.Lawrys.com
	www.LiptonBrisk.com
	www.LiptonT.com
	www.Mayo.com

Welchs

www.PeanutButter.com
www.Popsicle.com
www.Ragu.com
www.SlimFast.com
www.TakeControl.com
www.TasteYouLove.com
www.WishBone.com
www.Welchs.com

Notes

Notes

Notes

Notes